Workbook for

# Medical–Surgical Nursing Care

## Second Edition

Melissa Black
Deborah L. Stevenson

Karen M. Burke
Priscilla Lemone
Elaine L. Mohn-Brown

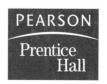

**PEARSON**

Prentice
Hall

Upper Saddle River, New Jersey 07458

Notice: Care has been taken to confirm the accuracy of the information presented in this book. The authors, editors, and the publisher, however, cannot accept any responsibility for errors or omissions or for consequences from application of the information in this book and make no warranty, express or implied, with respect to its contents.

The authors and the publisher have exerted every effort to ensure that drug selections and dosages set forth in this text are in accord with current recommendations and practice at time of publication. However, in view of ongoing research, changes in government regulations, and the constant flow of information relating to drug therapy and drug reactions, the reader is urged to check the package inserts of all drugs for any change in indications of dosage and for added warnings and precautions. This is particularly important when the recommended agent is a new and/or infrequently employed drug.

The authors and publisher disclaim all responsibility for any liability, loss, injury, or damage incurred as a consequence, directly or indirectly, of the use and application of any of the contents of this volume.

Pearson Education LTD.
Pearson Education Australia PTY, Limited
Pearson Education Singapore, Pte. Ltd
Pearson Education North Asia Ltd
Pearson Education, Canada, Ltd

Pearson Educación de Mexico, S.A. de C.V.
Pearson Education—Japan
Pearson Education Malaysia, Pte. Ltd
Pearson Education, Upper Saddle River, New Jersey

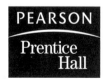

10   9   8   7   6   5   4   3   2   1
ISBN 0-13-188461-1

# Contents

# Preface

Students entering the field of nursing have a tremendous amount to learn in a short time. This Workbook that accompanies, *Medical–Surgical Nursing Care, 2/E* is designed to reinforce the knowledge that you—the student—has gained in each chapter and to help you master the critical concepts.

At the beginning of each chapter in this Workbook, you will find a MediaLink box. Just as in the main textbook, this box identifies for you all the specific media resources and activities available for that chapter on the CD-ROM, the main textbook and the Companion Website. You will find references to animations from the CD-ROM, and case studies and care plans from the Companion Website to help you visualize and comprehend difficult concepts. Chapter by chapter, this MediaLink box hones your critical thinking skills and enables you to apply concepts from the book into practice.

In addition, each chapter includes a variety of questions and activities to help you comprehend difficult concepts and reinforce basic knowledge gained from textbook reading assignments. Following is a list of features included in this edition that will enhance your learning experience:

- A short introductory paragraph summarizing the objective of each chapter.
- **Matching** exercise that contains key terms and definitions from each chapter.
- Thorough assessment of essential information in the text is provided through the **Fill in the Blank** activities.
- **Multiple Choice** questions that provide you with additional review on key topics.
- **Critical Thinking Activities** that apply concepts from the textbook to real nursing scenarios.
- **Answers** are included in the Appendix to provide immediate reinforcement and to permit you to check the accuracy of your work.

It is our hope that this Workbook will serve as a valuable learning tool and will contribute to your success in the nursing profession.

# Contributors

**Melissa Black, RN, MSN, FNP**
Greenville Technical College
Greenville, South Carolina

**Deborah Stevenson, RN, BSN**
Midland Technical College
Columbia, South Carolina

# Chapter 1

# The Medical–Surgical Nurse

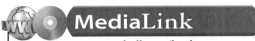

**MediaLink**

**www.prenhall.com/burke**

Use the address above to access the free, interactive Companion Website created for this textbook. Get hints, instant feedback, and textbook references to chapter-related NCLEX-style questions. Link to other interesting sites.

**Audio Glossary:**
Use the Companion Website, or the CD-ROM disk enclosed with your textbook, to hear the pronunciation of key terms in this chapter.

The medical–surgical nurse focuses on the client's responses to both actual and potential problems. The nursing process is utilized to assess, diagnose, plan, implement, and evaluate these responses. In addition, the nurse serves in the role of teacher and advocate.

## MEDICAL–SURGICAL TERMINOLOGY

Match each term with its appropriate definition.

1. _____ Caregiver
2. _____ Collaborate
3. _____ Caring
4. _____ Advocate
5. _____ NANDA
6. _____ Taxonomy
7. _____ Prioritization
8. _____ Documentation

9. _____ Critical thinking
10. _____ Ethics

A. The act of being concerned about something
B. Dealing with good and evil, moral principles
C. Listing items or actions in order of importance
D. One who represents and speaks for another
E. Develops nursing diagnoses
F. To work jointly with others
G. Classification system
H. Anyone who provides emotional or physical assistance
I. The act of writing facts
J. Using careful judgment in decision making

## FILL IN THE BLANK

Fill in the blanks with the appropriate word or phrase.

1. The LPN is aware that assuming responsibility for one's own actions, seeking additional learning experiences, and utilizing appropriate knowledge and skills are all examples of the National Association for Practical Nurse Education and Service's _____.

2. The _____ is a model of care that differentiates nursing practices from the practices of other health care providers.

3. The importance of interpersonal skills, adult learning principles, and therapeutic communication techniques are needed for the role of _____.

4. The quality control activities of evaluating, monitoring, or regulating the standards of service provided to the client are called _____.

5. The method of writing a nursing diagnosis most commonly used in nursing practice is _____.

6. A thorough history and physical that provides comprehensive data about a client is called the _____.

7. The American Nurses Association established a framework that states principles of ethical concern. First published in 1950, it guides the behavior of nurses and defines nursing for the general public. This document is referred to as the _____.

## MULTIPLE CHOICE

Circle the answer that best completes the following statements.

1. You overhear several students talking about a patient in the cafeteria. Knowing that this is a breach of confidentiality, the most appropriate action is to:
   A. do nothing.
   B. report the students to their clinical instructor.
   C. tactfully remind the students that they are breaking confidentiality rights.
   D. glare in the direction of the students.

2. A nurse has been assigned to care for an alert and oriented HIV client. The nurse states that she is afraid of contracting the virus. The charge nurse should:
   A. honor her wishes and give the client to someone else.
   B. remind her that nurses have a moral obligation to care for all persons.
   C. ignore the comment.
   D. discuss the nurse's fears with the director of nursing.

3. A client states that the pain medication is not working. After unsuccessfully attempting other alternative comfort measures, you notify the doctor. This is an example of a client:
   A. advocate.
   B. teacher.
   C. caregiver.
   D. care manager.

4. You are asked to review a client's chart to determine if an appropriate pain management regime was followed after a surgical procedure. This type of audit is known as:
   A. quality care.
   B. quality advocacy.
   C. quality assurance.
   D. quality concerns.

5. The charge nurse has asked you to gather data from the chart to assist in the development of a care plan. This phase of the nursing process is called:
   A. assessment.
   B. diagnosis.
   C. planning.
   D. evaluation.

6. A client who was admitted for a broken femur has now developed fever and chills. The nurse makes an assessment of the client's present condition. This type of data collection is called:
   A. initial.
   B. focused.
   C. late.
   D. inspection.

7. A client is experiencing shortness of breath, increased respirations, and profuse sweating. Which of these nursing diagnoses best defines the client's health problem?
   A. Ineffective Breathing Pattern
   B. Caregiver Role Strain
   C. Risk for Injury
   D. Chronic Pain

8. Your client has a temperature of 102°F and chills. Which response should the nursing diagnosis identify?
   A. potential problem
   B. actual problem
   C. new problem
   D. real problem

9. A 24-year-old male received severe neck injuries from a car wreck. He is on Demerol for pain. The nurse is developing a care plan based on the diagnosis of acute pain. Which of the following would be considered the etiology of this diagnosis?
   A. pain
   B. car wreck
   C. severe neck injuries
   D. Demerol

10. Mr. Johnson tells the nurse that he is nauseated and has vomited twice since breakfast. His vital signs are T-99, P-100, R-22, BP-142/74. These signs and symptoms are indicated by the phrase:
    A. as manifested by.
    B. as seen by.
    C. as noticed by.
    D. as revealed by.

11. Your client is recovering from hip surgery. You have decided that the best diagnosis for this client is Impaired Comfort. Which of the following have the responsibility to decide on a goal for this client?
    A. nurse
    B. nurse and client's significant other
    C. nurse and client
    D. nurse and caregiver

12. A client has the following goal: Client will walk down the hall by discharge. What part of the goal is missing?
    A. client
    B. time
    C. measurement
    D. Goal statement is complete.

13. The nurse identifies that a client is at risk for constipation. Which of the following would not be considered appropriate interventions?
    A. decrease water intake to four glasses per day
    B. ambulate t.i.d.
    C. administer a stool softener
    D. start an IV of $D_5W$ at 200 mL/hour as ordered

14. You are evaluating the following goal: Nursing assistant will demonstrate proper hand washing by the end of this lab session. Which of the following actions indicate that the goal has been met?
    A. Assistant rinses with cold water and wipes his hands on his shirt.
    B. Assistant turns off the water with his clean hands.
    C. Assistant removes rings prior to washing his hands.
    D. Assistant wipes hands on a damp paper towel.

15. Which of the following is not a component of critical thinking?
    A. sorting of relevant data
    B. defining a term and noting similarities and differences
    C. discriminating between facts and hunches
    D. making emergency decisions

## CRITICAL THINKING EXERCISE

Read the following situation. Unscramble the words and define each term. Answer the questions using the nursing process of assessment, diagnosis, planning, implementation, and evaluation.

A 78-year-old terminally ill client is refusing food and water. He has given the hospital an *dvdcanae tceredivi* and has named his son as a *rbaduel werpo fo turotaye.* As client *cvoteada,* the nurse must first review the legal documents and then proceed as directed.

The physician has ruled the client competent to make his own decisions. The son disagrees with his father's decision. This situation is referred to as an *tcalhie dmeamil.*

1. What are the two unpleasant alternatives in this situation?
2. Which of the client's rights is being questioned?
3. What vital information is missing from this case?
4. Why must the nurse document the problem?

# Chapter 2

# The Adult Client in Health and Illness

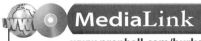

Effective nursing care begins with an understanding of the developmental stage of the client. The adult client comprises several stages. Each stage uniquely contributes to the ability of the client to cope with health and illness.

## ADULT BEHAVIORS AND MENTAL CONDITIONS

Match each term with its appropriate definition.

| | | | |
|---|---|---|---|
| 1. _____ | Alterations in health | A. | Diminished symptoms |
| 2. _____ | Gerontologic nursing | B. | State of reaching maximum health |
| 3. _____ | Family | C. | Individuals tied by marriage, birth, or adoption |
| 4. _____ | Couple | D. | Care of the older adult |
| 5. _____ | Health | E. | Signs and symptoms |
| 6. _____ | Wellness | F. | Reappearance of symptoms |
| 7. _____ | Manifestations | G. | Two people living together |
| 8. _____ | Illness | H. | State of complete mental, physical, and social well-being |
| 9. _____ | Remission | I. | A change from the normal wellness state |
| 10. _____ | Exacerbation | J. | Response to sickness |

## FILL IN THE BLANK

Fill in the blanks with the appropriate word or phrase.

1. An 18-year-old male is being counseled on the risk of contracting herpes. The nurse knows that this client would be considered in the developmental stage of _____.

2. Promoting the health of a 44-year-old female diagnosed with breast cancer is a major responsibility for the nurse. To communicate effectively, the nurse must understand the developmental stage of the _____.

3. You are correcting a nursing assistant who tells you that Mr. Cure is too old to learn how to change his wound dressing. You remind her that Mr. Cure may be 86 years old but can still learn. This adult stage is referred to as _____.

4. A client, age 65, tells you that she is concerned about the brown spots on her hands. You explain that these are normal aging processes for the adult stage of _____.

5. An 80-year-old client is preparing to be discharged to a nursing facility. You ask the charge nurse about the care he will receive. The nurse replies that the facility has a lot of experience caring for this age group. The age group that the charge nurse is referring to is _____.

6. Although accidents are the major cause of death in young adults, _____ ranks next and is the result of this age group's inability to cope with stress.

7. The development tasks of a family with adolescents and young adults generally focus on _____.

## MULTIPLE CHOICE

Circle the answer that best completes the following statements.

1. Which of the following behaviors would not be considered healthy for a young adult?
   A. eating hamburgers and French fries every day for lunch
   B. including 30 minutes of aerobic exercise three times a week
   C. decreasing the amount of sodas to one per day
   D. checking for breast lumps once a month

2. A 51-year-old male client asks his nurse what should be included in his routine physical examination. The most accurate response would be:
   A. barium enema every 2 years.
   B. PSA check annually.
   C. vision test every 6 months.
   D. stool for occult blood every 3 years.

3. You are assisting in the home inspection for a client recovering from a broken hip. Which of the following might require nursing teaching and intervention?
   A. throw rugs in two of the four rooms
   B. smoke alarm installed in the kitchen
   C. water temperature setting of warm
   D. handrails in the bathtub

4. You are assessing the physical condition of a 30-year-old male. You will not be surprised to find which of these signs and symptoms?
   A. full lung sounds
   B. heart rate of 68 bpm with maximum output
   C. smooth skin
   D. visual acuity of 20/30

5. A client in her middle adult years is concerned about her loss of inches in height. Your best reply should be:
   A. "It could be bone cancer, we should tell the doctor."
   B. "Loss of height is normal."
   C. "You are losing muscle mass, it just looks like you are getting shorter."
   D. "The vertebral discs may be thinning due to osteoporosis."

6. A client has developed a urinary tract infection due to the insertion of a Foley catheter. This type of illness is referred to as:
   A. functional.
   B. communicable.
   C. iatrogenic.
   D. acute.

7. Which of the following conditions would most likely be seen in the young adult?
   A. hypertension
   B. cardiovascular disease
   C. herpes
   D. obesity

8. The nurse is teaching a group of high school students about risks of respiratory diseases. He would be accurate if he said that the most common cause of lung problems is:
   A. smoking.
   B. inhalation of aerosols.
   C. working in a coal mine.
   D. breathing dust from the environment.

9. A young client is brought into the emergency room in a stupor. His friends say that he had broken up with his girl friend two nights ago and has been acting strange. The nurse suspects that this client has attempted:
   A. to get attention from his girlfriend.
   B. to kill himself.
   C. to fall asleep in order to forget the incident.
   D. to play a trick on his friends.

10. The nurse is aware that her client, a 46-year-old housewife, has overdosed on a medication. The nurse knows that the most common medication abused in this age group is:
    A. pain killers.
    B. sleeping pills.
    C. tranquilizers.
    D. antibiotics.

11. Which of the following is considered a family?
    A. father, mother, children, grandparents
    B. father, children, grandparents
    C. father, mother, grandparents
    D. all of the above

12. Which of the following may have an effect on an individual's perception of health?
    A. educational level
    B. cultural background
    C. developmental level
    D. all of the above

## CRITICAL THINKING EXERCISE

Read the following situation. Unscramble the words and define each term. Answer the questions using the nursing process of assessment, diagnosis, planning, implementation, and evaluation.

A 19-year-old female client has been diagnosed with *cutea* appendicitis. She is admitted to the surgical floor for IV therapy and possible appendectomy. In addition to this condition, the physician's note indicates *stancesub busae* of alcohol and a past history of *hogroaner*. He orders a *nancypegr* test. The nurse knows to observe for signs of alcohol withdrawal.

1. In this stage of illness, what behaviors might be observed in the client?
2. Discuss the risk factors that might have contributed to the gonorrhea and the physician's order for a pregnancy test.
3. Discuss the difference between an acute and chronic illness.
4. The pregnancy test comes back positive. What should the nurse document in the medical chart?

# Chapter 3

# The Older Adult Client in Health and Illness

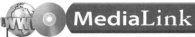

**MediaLink**

www.prenhall.com/burke

Use the address above to access the free, interactive Companion Website created for this textbook. Get hints, instant feedback, and textbook references to chapter-related NCLEX-style questions. Link to other interesting sites.

**Audio Glossary:**

Use the Companion Website, or the CD-ROM disk enclosed with your textbook, to hear the pronunciation of key terms in this chapter.

Physical and psychologic changes occur as individuals age. As the number of older Americans increases, nursing interventions and teaching must be designed to meet their specific needs.

## ADULT BEHAVIORS AND MENTAL CONDITIONS

Match each term with its appropriate definition.

1. _____ Aging
2. _____ Free radicals
3. _____ Apoptosis
4. _____ Havighurst
5. _____ Ageism
6. _____ Dementia

7. _____ Erikson
8. _____ Senescence theory
9. _____ Sundowning
10. _____ Kohlberg

A. Believed the major tasks of old age centered on maintaining social contacts and relationships

B. Term used to refer to different kinds of organic disorders

C. Unstable and reactive molecules

D. Identified ego integrity versus despair and disgust as the last stage of human development

E. Normal process occurring in cellular death

F. Believed older adults have completed the stages of moral development, and are at the conventional level

G. Form of prejudice against older adults

H. Focus on why people live as long as they do

I. Confusion that occurs after dark

J. Universal process beginning at birth

## FILL IN THE BLANK

Fill in the blanks with the appropriate word or phrase.

1. Aging is a normal process that begins at birth. The study of this process is called _____.

2. Mrs. Gary, an 87-year-old female, is diagnosed with uterine cancer. To communicate effectively, the nurse must understand the developmental stage of the _____.

3. You are teaching Mr. Woo, a 72-year-old male client, how to change his colostomy bag. This adult stage is referred to as _____.

4. A client, age 78, tells you that she is concerned about vaginal dryness during sex. You explain that these are normal aging processes for the adult stage of _____.

5. Based on the _____ a person has fewer defenses against foreign organisms as they age.

6. The current life expectancy in the United States is_____.

7. The average older adult has an average of 11 prescriptions filled per year. This predisposes them to adverse _____ and _____.

## MULTIPLE CHOICE

Circle the answer that best completes the following statements.

1. The nurse overhears a 76-year-old client's family member state, "Well he's had his good years, what can he possibly do to help us when he gets out?" This is a form of:
   A. genetic theory.
   B. apoptosis.
   C. ageism.
   D. senescence.

2. Calcium intake in older adults should average:
   A. 1200 mg per day.
   B. 600 mg per day.
   C. 800 mg per day.
   D. 1600 mg per day.

3. Older people continue to develop:
   A. judgmentally.
   B. cognitively.
   C. gerontonlogically.
   D. accidentally.

4. You are assessing the physical condition of an 80-year-old male. You will not be surprised to find which of these signs and symptoms?
   A. rales
   B. decreased skin turgor
   C. smooth skin
   D. visual acuity of 20/20

5. When making a home visit to your 66-year-old client, she states, "I made fried chicken and a peach cobbler yesterday. Would you care for some?" Your best reply should be:
   A. "Oh, no that's too much fat!"
   B. "Sure, where is the butter?"
   C. "I will send a dietician to discuss alternative cooking options."
   D. "Did you make collard greens also?"

6. The nurse is teaching the daughter of an elderly client about the aging process. The nurse would be correct if she stated:
   A. "Your father may develop an enlarged prostate."
   B. "Estrogen levels begin to increase in females as they get older."
   C. "Hypoglycemia is common in the elderly."
   D. "The infection risks are decreased due to the adrenal gland's enlargement."

7. Which of the following conditions would most likely be seen in the older adult?
   A. cataracts
   B. hypertension
   C. herpes
   D. obesity

8. You are talking to a client's son about the care his 78-year-old father will need at home. Your greatest concern for this client should be:
   A. Risk for Falls.
   B. Risk for Infection.
   C. Risk for Impaired Mobility.
   D. Risk for Caregiver Role Strain.

9. The nurse is aware that a family who takes care of a patient with Alzheimer's:
   A. realizes the disease is reversible.
   B. allows the patient to wander without constraint.
   C. may need the help of a support group.
   D. provides a stimulating environment.

10. Illness and loss of independence are:
    A. an expected part of the aging process.
    B. not inevitable.
    C. government issues.
    D. all of the above.

## CRITICAL THINKING EXERCISE

Read the following situation. Unscramble the words and define each term. Answer the questions using the nursing process of assessment, diagnosis, planning, implementation, and evaluation.

*Gagin* brings about *yscpialh* changes as well as the strong probability of *spycohcislao* changes. Nursing care promotes health in older adults and includes teaching healthy *vibrehosa* and encouraging healthy *fesyletlsi*.

1. Name five illnesses noted in older adulthood.
2. What nursing diagnoses go along with those illnesses?
3. Discuss healthy lifestyle and behavioral issues of the older adult.

# Chapter 4

## Settings of Care

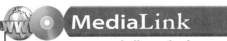
Community-based care allows for continuum of care extending from the acute care setting to the client's home. Nurses can use their expertise to facilitate the healing process by focusing on the individual and family health care needs.

## COMMUNITY CARE

Match each term with its appropriate definition.

| | | | |
|---|---|---|---|
| 1. _____ Client | | A. | Single largest reimbursement source |
| 2. _____ Community | | B. | Individual or family receiving services |
| 3. _____ OBRA | | C. | Regulates quality standards in long-term facilities |
| 4. _____ Home health agency | | D. | Process of learning to function with a disability |
| 5. _____ Rehabilitation | | E. | Provides care to clients who are unable to get it elsewhere |
| 6. _____ Clinic | | F. | Total adjustment to a disability within limits |
| 7. _____ Long-term care | | G. | Payment system based on diagnosis |
| 8. _____ Handicap | | H. | Organization that provides skilled home care |
| 9. _____ Medicare | | I. | Group of people living in the same region |
| 10. _____ DRGs | | J. | Provides care to clients who are unable to care for themselves |

## FILL IN THE BLANK

Fill in the blanks with the appropriate word or phrase.

1. Mrs. Anderson, 83 years old, has left-sided weakness as a result of a stroke 3 days ago. She requires maximum assistance for all of her ADLs. She

complains of pain and is upset about her inability to take care of herself and wants to go home. You suspect that the physician will order physical and occupational therapy so that Mrs. Anderson can begin the _____.

2. Mr. Jeffries calls your clinic with concerns about leaving his wife at home when he goes to work. Mrs. Jeffries suffers from mild confusion and, at times, has burned food on the stove due to forgetfulness. Mr. Jeffries is afraid that the house might catch on fire. He also tells you that his wife is able to manage her dressing, grooming, and toileting needs. Your best response would be to refer Mr. Jeffries to a(n) _____.

3. Adam, a 21-year-old male, was involved in a motorcycle accident 3 weeks ago. He tells you that the physician wants to discharge him directly to his home but he feels that he is not strong enough to walk without assistance. After discussing Adam's concerns with the physician, it is decided to place a request for _____.

4. You accompany the home health nurse to a client's home to assess the environment. You note that there are no handrails in the shower. In addition, there are several throw rugs on the floor in the living room. These issues are related to _____.

5. A 12-year-old patient has been diagnosed with osteosarcoma, a malignant tumor of the lower extremity. Amputation is the only treatment. This limitation of movement may be classified as a(n) _____.

6. A source document for managing home care and providing ethical guidelines for all home health clients is known as the _____.

7. A _____ is a person who recommends home health services and provides client-specific information needed for care.

## MULTIPLE CHOICE

Circle the answer that best completes the following statements.

1. A 70-year-old patient, recovering from a heart attack, continues to refuse to follow his ordered diet, take the appropriate medication, or attend the physical therapy sessions. You have been unable to motivate him. Your next action would be to:
   A. call his sister.
   B. call the patient advocate.
   C. set up a meeting with your supervisor and staff to discuss the issue.
   D. request a psychiatric consult from the physician.

2. Discharge planning should:
   A. be initiated after the client has met all treatment goals.
   B. begin when the care plan is initiated.
   C. include the family only if there is an order.
   D. start on admission to promote continuity of care.

3. Your patient, Mr. Hansen, is due to be discharged in 2 days. He insists that he will be going to his home. Your assessment reveals that Mr. Hansen requires maximum assistance with ADLs due to decreased range of motion as well as severe unsteadiness while attempting to walk. Your next action should be to:
    A. call the social worker to make arrangements for nursing home placement.
    B. call his family to schedule his time of discharge.
    C. tell the physician that a few more days in the hospital would be beneficial.
    D. coordinate a meeting with Mr. Hansen and family to discuss care needs.

4. Home health nurses must be resourceful and comfortable in their skills because:
    A. it is a difficult job.
    B. other nurses are not immediately available for consultation.
    C. caregiver burden can be destructive to the family unit.
    D. the patient will never see the doctor.

5. Mrs. Gutierrez is an 83-year-old with a new diagnosis of insulin-dependent diabetes mellitus. You are her home health nurse and are meeting her for the first time today. When you arrive she greets you suspiciously and quickly becomes angry. She wants to know how you plan to "run me and my life," then insists she doesn't need anyone. Your best response is:
    A. "I'm just here to help." Then begin teaching her about her disease.
    B. "If you want me to leave, I can come back later." Then set up a return visit.
    C. "I'm not here to run your life." Then ask her about her concerns.
    D. "What's your problem?" Then tell her to relax.

6. The current focus of care in hospitals is:
    A. caring for clients in the home setting.
    B. meeting the client's needs in a supervised setting.
    C. managing the general health of people in the community.
    D. treating the acutely ill and those needing surgery.

7. Community-based nursing focuses on:
    A. the health of the community.
    B. the culturally competent individual and family health care needs.
    C. getting people to use community resources instead of going to the hospital.
    D. rehabilitation of stroke victims and their families.

8. Home health care requires:
    A. doctor's orders.
    B. care plans.
    C. doctor's orders for evaluation and care.
    D. doctor's order for home health to begin and an approved treatment plan.

9. The amount of home health care services needed:
    A. increases with age.
    B. decreases with age.
    C. stays the same.
    D. has no relevance to age.

10. Home health nurses usually do not provide:
    A.  routine personal care.
    B.  medication administration.
    C.  wound care.
    D.  family teaching.

11. Older adults are increasingly moving to adult retirement centers. The focus of these centers is:
    A.  independence.
    B.  function.
    C.  security.
    D.  safety.

12. Diagnostic-related groups were introduced into the financing of health care to:
    A.  increase financial gains.
    B.  control costs.
    C.  provide hospitals with incentives to discharge clients.
    D.  regulate private practice of physicians.

13. In order to receive Medicare for home health care, the client must:
    A.  live alone.
    B.  exist at poverty level.
    C.  need help with cooking and cleaning.
    D.  all of the above.

14. Programs that provide recreation, meals, and social stimulation are referred to as:
    A.  long-term care facilities.
    B.  day care centers.
    C.  community clinics.
    D.  retirement centers.

15. The role of the home health nurse includes:
    A.  patient advocate.
    B.  care provider.
    C.  educator.
    D.  all of the above.

## CRITICAL THINKING EXERCISE

Read the following situation. Unscramble the words and define each term. Answer the questions using the nursing process of assessment, diagnosis, planning, implementation, and evaluation.

Mr. Elliot is a 72-year-old male who had a stroke 6 days ago. He has been stable for several days. He requires maximum assistance with ADLs and transfers. He is slow to process new information and has some residual expressive aphasia. He is to be discharged from the hospital to a *glonmetr race citylafi* for *nreoihtaatilbi* before returning to the *tummyconi*. While you are assisting him to the bathroom, he becomes loud and angry, stating, "I'm useless with this *tiprnaimme*. I'll never be whole again."

1. What assessment data should be gathered for Mr. Elliot's discharge?
2. What would you consider to be the most important data at this time?
3. Name the most appropriate nursing diagnosis for this client and list three nursing interventions.
4. Would the nurse document the statement, "Mr. Elliot is mad because he cannot move about like he used to" or "Mr. Elliot became loud and angry while being assisted to the bathroom. He stated: 'I'm useless with this impairment. I'll never be whole again'"? Explain your rationale.

# Chapter 5

## Guidelines for Client Assessment

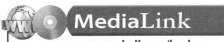

**www.prenhall.com/burke**

Use the address above to access the free, interactive Companion Website created for this textbook. Get hints, instant feedback, and textbook references to chapter-related NCLEX-style questions. Link to other interesting sites.

**Audio Glossary:**

Use the Companion Website, or the CD-ROM disk enclosed with your textbook, to hear the pronunciation of key terms in this chapter.

A complete and thorough assessment of the client is essential in order to provide effective, safe care. Assessment includes data collection based on the client's history and data collected during a physical examination. Documentation of the findings is vital in order to provide appropriate and effective nursing care.

## ASSESSMENT TECHNIQUES AND TERMS

Match each term with its appropriate definition.

1. _____ Inspection
2. _____ Palpation
3. _____ Percussion
4. _____ Auscultation
5. _____ Subjective data
6. _____ Objective data
7. _____ Primary source
8. _____ Secondary source
9. _____ Manifestations
10. _____ LOC

A. Sign, observable or measurable information
B. Tapping the body to produce sound waves
C. Client as information source
D. Observing/looking carefully
E. Symptoms experienced by the client
F. Listening to sounds using a stethoscope
G. Family, friends, or records as information sources
H. Objective and subjective data associated with an illness
I. Using the hands to touch and feel
J. Level of consciousness

## FILL IN THE BLANK

Fill in the blanks with the appropriate word or phrase.

1. The general survey provides information regarding the overall appearance and behavior of the client. Name ten items that should be assessed at this time: _____, _____, _____, _____, _____, _____, _____, _____, _____, _____.

2. An abnormal blue or gray discoloration of the skin due to decreased oxygen in the bloodstream is called _____.

3. A paleness of the skin related to blood loss is referred to as _____.

4. The normal pupil response to bright light is _____.

5. The _____ of the stethoscope is best for high-pitched sounds, such as $S_1$ and $S_2$.

6. The chart most often used for visual acuity is the _____ chart.

7. High-pitched sounds heard when air passes through narrowed bronchioles are called _____.

## MULTIPLE CHOICE

Circle the answer that best completes the following statements.

1. Poor turgor and dry mucous membranes would be an indication of:
   A. fluid volume deficit.
   B. fluid volume excess.
   C. normal fluid balance.
   D. not enough data to evaluate.

2. A grating sound heard during chest auscultation may be:
   A. crackles.
   B. pleural friction rub.
   C. rhonchi.
   D. wheezes.

3. Your client complains of difficulty breathing when attempting to lie down. After your respiratory assessment, you note in the medical record that the client has a history of:
   A. eupnea.
   B. apnea.
   C. orthopnea.
   D. dyspnea.

4. After the assessment of the eyes, the nurse would not document:
   A. equality.
   B. shape.
   C. reactivity.
   D. color of iris.

5. The normal pupillary response to accommodation is:
   A. dilatation and divergence.
   B. dilatation and convergence.
   C. constriction and divergence.
   D. constriction and convergence.

6. The use of adequate lighting is most important during:
   A. auscultation.
   B. percussion.
   C. palpation.
   D. inspection.

7. Ms. Lewis has a fractured tibia and fibula. The nurse is performing an assessment of her extremities. The purpose of the blanching test is to evaluate:
   A. peripheral circulation.
   B. cardiac output.
   C. peripheral pulses.
   D. nutritional deficiencies.

8. The student nurse is performing a cardiac assessment. You indicate your knowledge of the thoracic structures by properly palpating the PMI:
   A. directly over the sternum at the fourth rib.
   B. at the left midclavicular line, fifth intercostal space.
   C. at the right midclavicular line, fourth intercostal space.
   D. at the left midclavicular line, parallel to the axilla.

9. While assessing your client's lung fields, you hear popping sounds during inspiration at the base of the left lung. You would classify these findings as:
   A. crackles.
   B. rhonchi.
   C. wheezes.
   D. rubs.

10. An example of objective data would include:
   A. the client's description of the pain.
   B. radial pulse rate of 66 bpm.
   C. sensation of itching after a bee sting.
   D. headache resulting from photosensitivity.

11. A client states that he has had severe abdominal cramping for the last 2 hours. This type of data would be classified as an example of:
   A. subjective data.
   B. objective data.
   C. disputable data.
   D. personal data.

12. When assessing peripheral pulses, the nurse must compare both extremities. The elements of this assessment include:
    A. rate.
    B. rhythm.
    C. strength.
    D. all of the above.

13. The nurse prepares to assess the client's abdomen. The correct order of assessment should be:
    A. inspection, auscultation, palpation.
    B. inspection, palpation, auscultation.
    C. auscultation, inspection, palpation.
    D. any order is acceptable.

14. Mr. Hibbard has been admitted to the orthopedic unit following a motor vehicle collision. Both arms are placed in long-arm casts. When taking the vital signs, the nurse must assess the pulse rate by:
    A. listening to the apical pulse for one full minute.
    B. placing the client on a cardiac monitor.
    C. checking the carotid pulses.
    D. not assessing the radial pulses due to location of the cast.

15. The most accurate method for assessing the pulse rate is:
    A. simultaneous bilateral manipulation of the carotid arteries.
    B. auscultating directly over the point of maximum impulse.
    C. palpating the radial pulses.
    D. auscultating the femoral pulses.

## CRITICAL THINKING EXERCISE

Read the following situation. Unscramble the words and define each term. Answer the questions using the nursing process of assessment, diagnosis, planning, implementation, and evaluation.

The student nurse is caring for a client who was admitted 2 days ago with the diagnosis of left congestive heart failure. The nurse knows the *tatsifaneionsm* of this condition may include *dpsyean,* frothy sputum, and chest pain. An *ssssentmea* was performed at the beginning of the shift that included *pecinsnoit* and auscultation of the body systems. The client is now presenting with these classic symptoms in addition to a cough.

1. What type of assessment was performed at the beginning of the shift?
2. What type of assessment should be conducted at this time?
3. What data should be obtained immediately by the nurse?
4. Document your assessment findings.

# Chapter 6

## Essential Nursing Pharmacology

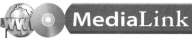

**www.prenhall.com/burke**

Use the address above to access the free, interactive Companion Website created for this textbook. Get hints, instant feedback, and textbook references to chapter-related NCLEX-style questions. Link to other interesting sites.

**Audio Glossary:**

Use the Companion Website, or the CD-ROM disk enclosed with your textbook, to hear the pronunciation of key terms in this chapter.

Medications are used to prevent disease, aid in the diagnosis and treatment of disease, and restore or maintain body system function. The nurse is responsible for understanding how medications affect their clients as well as the legal implications for administering medications.

## PHARMACOLOGY TERMINOLOGY

Match each term with its appropriate definition.

1. _____ Pharmacology     A.   Oral medication placed in the inner lining of the cheeks

2. _____ Pharmacokinetics     B.   The study of drugs and their uses in the body

3. _____ Absorption     C.   The process by which the body changes a drug from its original chemical structure to a form that can be readily eliminated or excreted

4. _____ Buccal     D.   Injectable drugs

5. _____ Parenteral     E.   Drugs that prevent a receptor response or block a normal cellular response

6. _____ Distribution     F.   Occurs after the drug has absorbed into the system

7. _____ Metabolism     G.   The process by which drugs are eliminated from the body

8. _____ Excretion     H.   The first step in the passage of a drug through the body

9. _____ Antagonist     I.   The amount of time needed for elimination processes to decrease the original blood concentration

10. _____ Half-life     J.   The study of how drugs are processed by the body

## FILL IN THE BLANK

Fill in the blanks with the appropriate word or phrase.

1. Mr. Wills is brought to the ED with active seizures. It is determined through labs that his Dilantin level is below therapeutic range. You know that the doctor will order a _____ of phenytoin to reach therapeutic drug levels rapidly.

2. Mrs. Smith's pain level was an 8 on a scale of 0–10 an hour ago. She was given morphine 8 mg IM and states, "I hardly have any pain, maybe a one if I move around," This is an example of drug _____ because the morphine has controlled her pain.

3. Asian clients may require a lower concentration of antianxiety medications. This is an example of how _____ plays a role in drug response.

4. When two drugs given together cause a greater response than each drug given separately, this is called _____.

5. The nurse knows that _____ occurs when Demerol and Phenergan are given together.

6. In 1938 the _____ added new regulations regarding labeling and packaging of drugs as well as requiring drug companies to perform toxicity tests on lab animals.

7. The _____ of 1970 identifies and regulates the manufacture and sale of narcotics and dangerous drugs.

## MULTIPLE CHOICE

Circle the answer that best completes the following statements.

1. All health care facilities are required to have narcotic control systems in place (i.e., all narcotics are locked up). One way of insuring compliance is to:
   A. give narcotic keys to all employees.
   B. give narcotic keys to administrative staff only.
   C. give narcotic keys to authorized personnel.
   D. not enough data to evaluate.

2. The most widely used drug reference in the United States is:
   A. hospital formulary.
   B. Facts and Comparisons.
   C. PSA.
   D. PDR.

3. The absorption process occurs from the time a drug enters the body until:
   A. it reaches the site of action.
   B. half-life is achieved.
   C. excretion.
   D. it quits working.

4. Transdermal (applied to the skin) patches absorb drugs slowly into the body and usually:
   A. last longer.
   B. fall off easily.
   C. cause rashes.
   D. provide relief.

5. Intravenous drugs are delivered directly into the bloodstream and therefore:
   A. have the slowest excretion rate.
   B. have the fastest absorption rate.
   C. have the greatest half-life.
   D. have the longest duration of action.

6. The blood–brain barrier protects the central nervous system against severe toxic drug effects by preventing access to the:
   A. spinal fluid.
   B. cerebrospinal fluid.
   C. synovial fluid.
   D. pleural cavity.

7. Drug metabolism refers to the process by which the body changes a drug from its original chemical structure to a form that can be readily eliminated or excreted. This is also called:
   A. biochemistry.
   B. bionics.
   C. biotransformation.
   D. bioefficiency.

8. Drug toxicity in older adults occurs as a result of
   A. ageism.
   B. negligence.
   C. confusion.
   D. polypharmacy.

9. The effect of a drug depends on its:
   A. type and client.
   B. time and route.
   C. action and dose.
   D. cost and manufacturer.

10. The nurse knows to include in her teaching:
    A. teas bind with tetracycline.
    B. a high carbohydrate diet decreases absorption of levodopa.
    C. a diet high in vitamin K reduces the effect of Coumadin.
    D. a diet low in protein delays the effect of theophylline.

## CRITICAL THINKING EXERCISE

Read the following situation. Unscramble the words and define each term. Answer the questions using the nursing process of assessment, diagnosis, planning, implementation, and evaluation.

There are different types of drug orders directing when the nurse should *mriainsrtde* drugs. A *gisatndn* order is used for a specific condition. Stat orders are done immediately. PRN orders are implemented when the client needs the drug, and routine orders are applied until a discontinuation order is written.

1. Name the six rights of drug administration.

2. Discuss the National Coordinating Council for Medication Error Reporting and Preventions' definition of a medication error. What are the most common errors that cause client death?

3. What strategy developed by the Joint Commission on Accreditation of Hospital Organizations (JCAHO) helps prevent medication errors?

# Chapter 7

## Caring for Clients with Altered Fluid, Electrolyte, or Acid–Base Balance

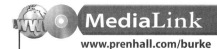

**MediaLink**

**www.prenhall.com/burke**

Use the address above to access the free, interactive Companion Website created for this textbook. Get hints, instant feedback, and textbook references to chapter-related NCLEX-style questions. Link to other interesting sites.

**Audio Glossary:**

Use the Companion Website, or the CD-ROM disk enclosed with your textbook, to hear the pronunciation of key terms in this chapter.

Fluids and electrolytes are in a delicate and complex balance within the body. Electrolytes aid in the maintenance of water balance, electrical impulses, cardiac rhythms, and bone formation. Water is vital for life and is the main component of body weight composition. Multiple body systems are on constant alert to detect and correct imbalances.

## FLUIDS AND ELECTROLYTES

Match each term with its appropriate definition.

1. _____ Thirst
2. _____ Intracellular fluid
3. _____ Sodium
4. _____ Extracellular fluid
5. _____ Hypertonic
6. _____ Osmolality
7. _____ Interstitial fluid
8. _____ Potassium
9. _____ Kidneys
10. _____ Fluid volume deficit

A. Primary regulator of water and electrolytes
B. Commonly caused by diarrhea or vomiting
C. Primary ECF cation
D. Higher concentration of solutes than plasma
E. Fluid found outside the cells
F. Fluid found between the cells
G. Concentration of all solutes within body fluid
H. Fluid found inside the cells
I. Primary indicator for regulation of water intake
J. Primary ICF cation

## FILL IN THE BLANK

Fill in the blanks with the appropriate word or phrase.

1. A client has just been admitted from the ER. His symptoms include nausea/vomiting, diarrhea, cardiac dysrhythmias, and numbness/tingling in the fingers and around the mouth. The nurse suspects that the patient may be diagnosed with _____.

2. Mr. Jones complains of a headache, muscle weakness, fatigue, apathy, and abdominal cramps. During your assessment, the client experiences postural hypotension. You suspect that Mr. Jones has an electrolyte imbalance known as _____.

3. An 89-year-old female is brought to your clinic by her daughter. Your assessment reveals muscle spasm and tetany. The 12-lead EKG shows significant cardiac irregularities. You suspect that this client may be experiencing _____.

4. Amy is a 3-year-old child suffering from cystic fibrosis. Due to chronic fluid in her lungs, she is having SOB. When checking her recent laboratory values you note an elevated $PaCO_2$ and bicarbonate blood level. Her lab studies reveal that this has been a chronic problem. You know that these high elevations are most likely due to _____.

5. Yesterday a 36-year-old male was admitted to your unit. He has a history of IDDM and renal insufficiency. Today he is lethargic and complaining of nausea. His lab shows an elevated potassium level. You suspect that this client has an abnormal acid–base balance known as _____.

6. Mr. Wilson was admitted 3 days ago for gastric surgery and has been on intermittent NG suctioning due to severe nausea. His vital signs are T-99, P-92, R-10, BP-130/62. On today's lab work you note a pH of 7.6, bicarbonate level of 27, and potassium level of 3.4. You know, based on this information, that the acid–base imbalance is probably _____.

7. A client is admitted to your medical floor with a diagnosis of pancreatitis and a history of CHF. His current medications are Lasix, digoxin, and vancomycin. Due to his physical condition and medications, you will monitor any neuromuscular changes that could indicate the development of _____.

## MULTIPLE CHOICE

Circle the answer that best completes the following statements.

1. The primary electrolyte that controls the water balance in the body is:
   A. sodium.
   B. potassium.
   C. chloride.
   D. magnesium.

2. Which of the following clients would be considered at greatest risk for dehydration?
   A. overweight male.
   B. average-weight male.
   C. underweight female.
   D. overweight female.

3. Of the following, which is not considered a function of an electrolyte?
   A. regulate acid–base balance.
   B. needed for nutritional value.
   C. maintain neuromuscular activity.
   D. assist with enzyme reactions.

4. Osmosis is the movement of:
   A. particles across a semipermeable membrane.
   B. water from an area of low-solute concentration to an area of higher concentration.
   C. water and solutes across the capillary membranes.
   D. solutes from an area of low concentration to an area of higher concentration.

5. Active transport is defined as:
   A. an example of a sodium-potassium pump.
   B. the movement of molecules from an area of low-solute concentration to an area of high-solute concentration via the ATP mechanism.
   C. cells in a constant state of motion.
   D. molecules that continually move in and out of cells.

6. Mr. Smith has recently been diagnosed with a kidney dysfunction. He constantly complains of thirst. Which of the following statements to the client best indicates the nurse's understanding of the thirst mechanism?
   A. "Thirst is the primary regulator of water intake. When we are thirsty, we drink."
   B. "It is important in maintaining fluid balance and preventing dehydration."
   C. "Thirst mechanisms decline with age, making the older adult at risk for dehydration."
   D. "A drop in blood volume stimulates the thirst center in the brain, which produces the sensation of 'thirst.'"

7. The mechanism of action for the antidiuretic hormone (ADH) may be defined as:
   A. kidneys reabsorb more water when the hormone is present.
   B. kidneys cease urine production when the hormone is present.
   C. blood osmolality increases as urine output decreases.
   D. the hypothalamus detects increased osmolality of the blood and stimulates the release of ADH.

8. The pathophysiology of SIADH is described as:
   A. a failure of the hypothalamus to release antidiuretic hormone.
   B. an excess of antidiuretic hormone in the bloodstream.
   C. water retention.
   D. copious amounts of concentrated urine.

9. Diabetes insipidus is caused by:
   A. failure of the hypothalamus to release antidiuretic hormone, resulting in excessive amounts of dilute urine.
   B. failure of the hypothalamus to release antidiuretic hormone, resulting in concentrated urine.
   C. failure of the pancreas to produce insulin, resulting in polyuria.
   D. total absence of antidiuretic hormone, resulting in severe water retention.

10. Alice is a 2-year-old child who has been suffering from vomiting and diarrhea for 3 days. Temperature is 102°F and she appears lethargic and exhausted. Her mother reports that Alice has not been able to keep anything down. Based on this information, Alice's primary nursing diagnosis should be:
    A. Activity Intolerance.
    B. Fluid Volume Deficit.
    C. Nutrition Altered: Less than Body Requirements.
    D. Risk for Diarrhea.

11. Your client has been admitted for uncontrollable vomiting. The doctor has ordered a Foley catheter and an IV of $D_5$ $\frac{1}{2}$ NS at 75 mL/hr. After the Foley was inserted, the initial amount of urine obtained was 100 mL. The IV was successfully begun, but 1 hour later the client's Foley bag had only drained 50 mL. Your next action would be to:
    A. administer an antiemetic in an attempt to stop the loss of gastric fluid.
    B. call the doctor and report the low urine output.
    C. continue to monitor.
    D. encourage the client to increase PO fluids.

12. Which electrolyte is most readily excreted by the kidneys and will be lost even when other electrolytes are conserved?
    A. potassium
    B. sodium
    C. magnesium
    D. calcium

13. Which of the following statements is false regarding the acid–base balance system?
    A. Blood buffers react quickly but are limited.
    B. The respiratory system adjusts the acid–base balance by either slowing or increasing respirations.
    C. The renal system is the slowest of the systems but is responsible for long-term balance.
    D. When hydrogen ions and the pH in the blood increase, the result is acidosis.

14. A patient suffering from metabolic acidosis is most likely to:
    A. experience an increase in the blood pH.
    B. develop tachypnea.
    C. recover slowly, due to the kidney's role in acid–base balance.
    D. be diagnosed with acute pneumonia.

15. Mr. Jacobs, who was diagnosed with COPD 5 years ago, has been using his oxygen at home via nasal cannula. The flow rate is set at 2 L/min. Mr. Jacobs' respirations are 28/min, and he complains of SOB after minimal exertion. His wife is concerned that the amount of oxygen is "too low." Your best response should be:
    A.  "I can't change the flow rate without an order."
    B.  "Okay, let's increase the flow rate to 6 L/min and see how he does."
    C.  "Increasing his oxygen may actually cut off his respiratory center in the brain."
    D.  "I'll call the doctor and let him know about your concerns."

## CRITICAL THINKING EXERCISE

Read the following situation. Unscramble the words and define each term. Answer the questions using the nursing process of assessment, diagnosis, planning, implementation and evaluation.

A 73-year-old female is admitted for *poolymihave* related to severe nausea, vomiting, and diarrhea. The physician diagnoses her with *metryhpoinaa* and *amilyahokpe*. He orders IV fluid of $D_5$ ½ NS at 125 mL/hr to help correct her *rolceeltyet* imbalance. Two days later, she begins to complain of SOB and chest discomfort. You suspect that this client has now developed fluid overload.

1.  What is your primary nursing intervention at this time?
2.  What factors have contributed to her condition?
3.  What orders do you expect will be written in the chart?
4.  How would you document these assessment findings?

# Chapter 8

## Caring for Clients in Pain

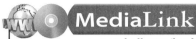

**MediaLink**

**www.prenhall.com/burke**

Use the address above to access the free, interactive Companion Website created for this textbook. Get hints, instant feedback, and textbook references to chapter-related NCLEX-style questions. Link to other interesting sites.

**Audio Glossary:**

Use the Companion Website, or the CD-ROM disk enclosed with your textbook, to hear the pronunciation of key terms in this chapter.

Pain can be caused by physiologic as well as emotional stressors. Pain is subjective. The idea that "perception is reality" is the cornerstone of pain management. The nurse must accept what the patient states as fact. A thorough assessment and plan of care for the client in pain is the nurse's priority.

## PAIN TERMINOLOGY

Match each term with its appropriate definition.

| | | |
|---|---|---|
| 1. _____ Pain | A. | Can be given alone for moderate-to-severe pain |
| 2. _____ Analgesia | B. | Seeking of drugs for nonmedical reasons |
| 3. _____ Perception | C. | Amount of pain endured before seeking relief |
| 4. _____ Opioids | D. | Patient-controlled analgesia |
| 5. _____ Pain threshold | E. | Unpleasant sensory or emotional experience |
| 6. _____ Respiratory depression | F. | Point at which a person recognizes pain |
| 7. _____ PCA | G. | Antidote for opioids |
| 8. _____ Addiction | H. | Processing of pain impulses in the brain |
| 9. _____ Pain tolerance | I. | Major side effect of most narcotics |
| 10. _____ Narcan | J. | Pain relief |

## FILL IN THE BLANK

Fill in the blanks with the appropriate word or phrase.

1. Mr. Alexander calls the doctor's office where you work and tells you that he twisted his ankle a couple of days ago. He has been taking the medication that was prescribed but would like some suggestions on increasing his comfort. A nonpharmacologic intervention that might be suggested is to apply _____.

2. A patient states that he has never received so much attention before he was injured. He tells you that his pain actually provided many visitors and gifts. Later in the shift you notice that he starts moaning whenever he sees someone he knows. The perception that pain is a positive thing and will bring satisfaction is known as _____.

3. A client with severe sunburn on his back and arms is seen in your clinic. He describes the pain as sharp and burning. This type of pain is called _____.

4. A young woman with uncontrolled diabetes mellitus complains of a burning and tingling sensation in her feet and lower legs. This type of pain is called _____.

5. Mr. Fenogloi is a young executive with a history of hypertension. He presents to the emergency room with the following vital signs: T-99.1, P-110, R-24, BP-210/120. He is diaphoretic and states his chest is going to explode. The physician suspects Mr. Fenogloi has angina. Angina is caused by _____.

6. Mr. Beauchamp comes to your office complaining of an upset stomach. He tells you that the ibuprofen is making his stomach burn. The nurse should ask Mr. Beauchamp if he is taking the medication with _____ or _____.

7. A patient with severe cancer pain is most likely to be ordered an _____ for pain relief.

## MULTIPLE CHOICE

Circle the answer that best completes the following statements.

1. Natalie, a 26-year-old college student, has been admitted to your unit for observation. She has recently been found crying frequently alone in her room. She admits that she is constantly tired and irritable. The medical history reveals that Natalie was injured in a car accident 2 years ago and that she has never fully recovered. Natalie states that her back never stops hurting. You suspect that this may be diagnosed as:
   A. chronic pain syndrome.
   B. acute pain syndrome.
   C. chronic malignant pain.
   D. psychosomatic pain.

2. The nurse is caring for a client who received multiple fractures and contusions from a fall 5 days ago. At 3:30 P.M., the nurse administers the pain medication that was ordered q.i.d. At 5:00 P.M., the client calls for more pain medication. The assessment shows a BP of 160/88 and a pulse of 100. The nurse checks the chart and discovers that the client has made constant requests for pain relief on the previous shift. The best response would be to:
   A. ignore the client, as it appears he may be addicted to the medication.
   B. call the physician and report the addiction.
   C. administer another dose at 7:00 P.M.
   D. notify the physician that the current medication may not be effective.

3. Mrs. Hamrick is recovering from knee replacement surgery. Her pain medication order reads as follows: Vicodin 5/500 mg tabs 2 PO q.i.d. prn pain. She is scheduled for physical therapy from 10 to 11 A.M. It is now 7 A.M. She has not received a tab since 3 A.M. You will expect to administer the medication:
   A. at 9:30 A.M.
   B. at 10 A.M.
   C. after she returns from therapy.
   D. as soon as she calls for the medication.

4. Timothy, a 10-year-old, has twisted his ankle playing baseball. His mom asks you what other methods could be used to control the pain if the ordered medication does not work. You suggest:
   A. bring Timothy back to the clinic.
   B. place ice packs on the ankle for 20 minutes at a time for 24 hours.
   C. double the medication dosage.
   D. place warm packs on the ankle continuously for 24 hours.

5. A 70-year-old patient with a history of Parkinson's disease and arthritis has been placed on Darvocet N100 1 tab PO t.i.d. prn pain. Which of the following would be a priority nursing diagnosis?
   A. Constipation
   B. Disturbed Thought Processes
   C. Risk for Injury
   D. Activity Intolerance

6. Your client requires discharge teaching regarding his pain medication, Demerol tabs. Which of the following would be considered your highest priority?
   A. Do not take with alcohol.
   B. Constipation may occur.
   C. Sleepiness is a common side effect.
   D. Nausea can be decreased by taking with food.

7. Mrs. Johnnie has been ordered a PCA pump for pain control after her colon surgery. She voices concern about the potential for overdosing. Your best reply would be:
   A. "Don't worry, that never happens."
   B. "The pump is preset and you will only be allowed to receive that amount."
   C. "I'll teach you to use the pump and regulate the amount that you get."
   D. "If you are worried about it, we can give you injections instead."

8. A patient has been receiving a new pain medication every 4 hours as ordered. His wife is concerned that he is very sleepy all the time and may be overmedicated. Your best response would be:
   A. "It really is strange that he is that sleepy."
   B. "I'll call the doctor. Thanks for telling me."
   C. "It is not unexpected with a new pain medication. We are checking him every two hours."
   D. "If he doesn't wake up in four hours, we'll get the medication changed."

9. You receive a call from a patient who has been on long-term pain medications. She is worried that the pharmacist gave her "cheap stuff" because it does not help her pain. The patient may be developing:
   A. increased pain.
   B. tolerance to the medication.
   C. decreased pain tolerance.
   D. chronic pain.

10. Mrs. Wesley is at the doctor's office for a checkup. She asks you why the doctor would prescribe an antidepressant when she is complaining of pain. She says, "I'm not crazy, my back has just hurt for so long." You base your response on the fact that:
    A. antidepressants are capable of relieving many types of pain.
    B. pain can cause confusion.
    C. chronic pain can affect mood and sleep patterns.
    D. opioids work best when taken with other medications.

11. A 17-year-old boy was admitted to the emergency department for fractures received during a football game. He is moaning and crying. After watching you administer a shot of Demerol, the father asks, "Why is my son acting like a baby? He's never acted like this before when a bone was broken!" Your response is based on the fact that:
    A. everyone perceives pain differently.
    B. everyone has a different pain threshold.
    C. previous experiences with pain can affect future coping behaviors.
    D. all of the above.

12. The tool used to measure pain is called a:
    A. Pain Tolerance Guide.
    B. Pain Threshold Scale.
    C. Pain Conduction Tool.
    D. Pain Scale.

13. Increased blood pressure, dilated pupils, perspiration, and pallor are signs of:
    A. opiate overdose.
    B. acute pain.
    C. adverse effects of Demerol.
    D. chronic pain.

14. Chronic nonmalignant pain is:
    A. known as cancer pain.
    B. due to back pain.
    C. ongoing pain caused by non–life-threatening causes.
    D. ongoing pain caused by a malignant tumor.

15. Response to pain is affected by:
    A. family and cultural expectations.
    B. pain tolerance.
    C. past experiences with pain.
    D. all of the above.

## CRITICAL THINKING EXERCISE

Read the following situation. Unscramble the words and define each term. Answer the questions using the nursing process of assessment, diagnosis, planning, implementation, and evaluation.

Mrs. Smith is a cancer patient being admitted for treatment with chemotherapy. During the assessment, Mrs. Smith states that her pain is currently controlled by using a *ragesicDu nsmalerdrta* patch and several *xatoinlaer* techniques. During the course of her therapy, the physician places Mrs. Smith on a *tientpa llednoctro analaiseg* pump.

Two hours after initiating the pump, Mrs. Smith becomes very sleepy. Her respirations are 16/min. Three hours later, you are unable to wake Mrs. Smith. Her respirations are now 8/min and shallow.

1. What would be your next action in this situation?
2. What intervention would be provided by the registered nurse?
3. Discuss your nursing interventions while Mrs. Smith is recovering.
4. Document this incident in the nurse's notes.

# Chapter 9

# Caring for Clients Having Surgery

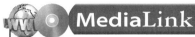

Surgery is an invasive medical procedure performed to diagnose, treat, or cure illness, injury, or deformity. The nurse assumes an active role in caring for the client before, during, and after surgery.

## SURGICAL TERMINOLOGY

Match each term with its appropriate definition.

1. _____ Conscious sedation
2. _____ General anesthesia
3. _____ Postoperative phase
4. _____ Emancipated minor
5. _____ Dehiscence
6. _____ Informed consent
7. _____ Secondary intention
8. _____ Regional anesthesia
9. _____ Intraoperative phase
10. _____ Evisceration

A. Begins with entry into the operating room
B. Local anesthesia
C. Operative permit
D. Protrusion of body organs from a wound
E. Provides analgesia/amnesia with wakefulness
F. Large, gaping, irregular wound
G. Separation of incisional wound
H. Under age 18, lives independently
I. Begins with admittance to recovery area
J. Unconsciousness state

## FILL IN THE BLANK

Fill in the blanks with the appropriate word or phrase.

1. This phase begins when the decision for surgery is made and ends when the client is transferred to the operating room: _____.

2. Breathing exercises taught to the client who may be at risk for developing postoperative pulmonary complications are called _____.

3. Two commonly used wound suction devices that promote drainage of fluid from an incision site are the _____ and _____ drains.

4. The trade name for diazepam is _____.

5. A position used for GYN, perineal, or rectal surgery is the _____ position.

6. A type of scrub performed to render hands and arms as clean as possible in preparation for a sterile procedure is referred to as a(n) _____.

7. Drainage that contains serum and red blood cells is called _____.

## MULTIPLE CHOICE

Circle the answer that best completes the following statements.

1. The nurse should know that the client's surgery will be postponed if the hemoglobin level is below:
   A. 16 g per 100 mL.
   B. 10 g per 100 mL.
   C. 12 g per 100 mL.
   D. 14 g per 100 mL.

2. A diabetic client is more at risk for postoperative complications because:
   A. the prescribed diet cannot be consumed due to nausea.
   B. healing rarely takes place in the diabetic client.
   C. blood glucose levels can fluctuate uncontrollably.
   D. the client is unable to administer self-injections of insulin.

3. Preoperative medications must be administered:
   A. within 15 minutes of the ordered time.
   B. within 30 minutes of the ordered time.
   C. at the ordered time.
   D. after the skin scrub is completed.

4. While the surgical client is semiconscious and receiving IV therapy, the nurse should:
   A. keep the arms unrestrained so the joints will not stiffen.
   B. elevate the arm above the level of the heart.
   C. gently massage the arm to relieve muscle spasms and prevent clots from forming.
   D. monitor the IV site at frequent intervals.

5. Immediately following surgery, the client's vital signs must be checked every:
   A. 5 minutes.
   B. 15 minutes.
   C. 20 minutes.
   D. 30 minutes.

6. Your client calls you to his room and tells you that something is wrong with his incision. You notice that the edges of the wound have separated and a small amount of beefy red tissue is observable. Your first response should be to:
    A. notify the physician.
    B. cover the wound with sterile dry dressing.
    C. place a normal saline sterile dressing over the wound.
    D. ask the client how long ago this occurred.

7. The nurse will instruct the client receiving a local anesthetic that:
    A. no pain will be felt during the procedure.
    B. drowsiness is a side effect of the medication.
    C. bleeding is usually superficial.
    D. consciousness will be lost.

8. The nurse should teach the client that, after surgery, DVT may be prevented by:
    A. raising the head of the bed.
    B. encouraging passive and active leg exercises.
    C. keeping the knees elevated.
    D. encouraging coughing and deep breathing exercises.

9. Which of the following is at a greater risk for developing postsurgical and postanesthesia complications?
    A. 42-year-old scheduled for eye surgery
    B. 3-year-old scheduled for a hernia repair
    C. 80-year-old scheduled for a right hip replacement
    D. 18-year-old scheduled for a cervical biopsy

10. You are asked to obtain an informed consent for a client who is scheduled for a bowel resection. Your main responsibility should be to:
    A. explain the risks involved with the surgery.
    B. discuss other medical options that might be useful for this client's condition.
    C. witness the client's signature of consent.
    D. check the form for completeness.

11. Your client is scheduled for surgery in 2 hours. He asks you why the surgery has to be done right away. He insists on a detailed explanation of the procedure. The legal responsibility for explaining the procedure rests with the:
    A. charge nurse.
    B. hospital risk management team.
    C. physician who will perform the surgery.
    D. patient advocate.

12. Coughing and deep breathing are techniques that must be taught to surgical patients to prevent:
    A. formation of clots at the incision site.
    B. lung collapse after the surgery.
    C. hypotension.
    D. prolonged pain.

13. Morphine and Demerol may be ordered as a preoperative medication to:
    A. eliminate spasms of the colon.
    B. enhance the effects of the anesthetic.
    C. decrease hypertensive episodes during surgery.
    D. reduce pain while in the recovery room.

14. It is important for the nurse to assess the client's home medications prior to surgery because:
    A. these medications may alter the client's perception of the surgery.
    B. the anesthetics received in the operative phase may cause toxicity of other drugs.
    C. some medications may interact with the anesthetics, causing undesired effects.
    D. routine medications are usually withheld the day of the surgery.

15. Mr. James is complaining of abdominal discomfort 2 days after his hernia repair. He tells you that he feels bloated and has no appetite. Your next action should be to:
    A. tell the client that this is normal and to ambulate as much as possible.
    B. ask Mr. James about his last bowel movement.
    C. assess bowel function.
    D. administer a stool softener.

## CRITICAL THINKING EXERCISE

Read the following situation. Unscramble the words and define each term. Answer the questions using the nursing process of assessment, diagnosis, planning, implementation, and evaluation.

Mrs. Lilly Fields is recovering from the effects of the *thsseianea* she received during surgery. You receive a report from the PACU nurse, who tells you that Mrs. Field is doing well. Vital signs are stable. A *ackonsJ ttraP* drain is located in the wound and is draining *sguinnauoes* fluid. Mrs. Fields is a chronic smoker and is at risk for *eleatsistac*. During your physical assessment you observe that she is moaning occasionally. She is drowsy but appears agitated and restless. Her pain is on a scale of 7. Her last dose of morphine was 1 hour ago. The medication order reads as follows: morphine 5–10 mg IM q3 hrs prn pain.

1. What nonverbal signs of pain does Mrs. Fields exhibit?
2. How would you document Mrs. Fields' pain?
3. What action should you take to relieve this client's discomfort?
4. Name one nursing diagnosis that would be appropriate for Mrs. Fields.

# Chapter 10

## Caring for Clients with Inflammation and Infection

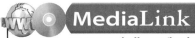

**MediaLink**

www.prenhall.com/burke

Use the address above to access the free, interactive Companion Website created for this textbook. Get hints, instant feedback, and textbook references to chapter-related NCLEX-style questions. Link to other interesting sites.

**Audio Glossary:**

Use the Companion Website, or the CD-ROM disk enclosed with your textbook, to hear the pronunciation of key terms in this chapter.

The immune system is designed to fight infection and heal injuries in the body. Inflammation is the first response to infection or injury. Infection occurs only after a chain of events takes place. If any of these links are broken, infection cannot occur.

## ANATOMY AND PHYSIOLOGY

Match each term with its appropriate definition.

1. _____ Macrophage
2. _____ Phagocytosis
3. _____ Lymphadenitis
4. _____ Leukocytosis
5. _____ Skin
6. _____ Mucous membranes
7. _____ Cilia
8. _____ Urine
9. _____ Gastric fluid
10. _____ Endogenous pyrogens

A. First line of defense against external organisms
B. Removes trapped microorganisms from respiratory tract
C. Chemicals released by macrophages that cause fever
D. Washes away microorganisms
E. Lines the inner surfaces of the mouth and nose
F. Large WBC that ingest microorganisms and dead tissue
G. A systemic response to inflammation
H. Increased WBC production
I. The ingestion of microorganisms and dead tissue
J. Contains bactericidal substances

## FILL IN THE BLANK

Fill in the blanks with the appropriate word or phrase.

1. A 24-year-old man hobbles into your clinic with complaints of a painful, swollen ankle received from a fall 2 days ago. During your assessment, you find out the client saw a physician who stated that the ankle was not broken. The client is in your clinic because he is concerned about the continued swelling and pain in his ankle. You recognize the client is continuing to experience _____ inflammation.

2. A 40-year-old woman has presented in your clinic for complaints of a sore throat and fatigue. Vital signs are T-102, BP-124/82, P-96, R-20. Upon palpation of her neck, you note swollen lymph nodes. The physician orders a WBC count and throat culture. The lab results indicate elevated WBCs. Based on these findings you understand the client is demonstrating _____ of acute inflammation.

3. You are caring for an elderly woman who has arthritis. She takes corticosteroids to manage the pain in her joints. She tells you she has been having pain and swelling in her joints for about 10 years. You understand this pain and swelling is related to _____ inflammation.

4. A client complains of fatigue, fever, sore throat, and decreased appetite. The physician has ordered a WBC count with differential. You understand the physician will use the differential to decide on the type of _____.

5. You are working in a pediatrician's office and receive a phone call from the mother of a child you saw several days ago who was treated for strep throat. The mother is concerned that her child may still be contagious to others. Upon questioning the mother, you find out the child's fever is gone, his sore throat has diminished, and he has been taking antibiotics for 3 days. You reply that her child is not contagious any longer. This reply is based on your knowledge of the stages of the infectious process, and that this child is in the _____ stage.

6. You are caring for a client in a hospital who had surgery for a broken leg. After the surgery, your client developed a distended bladder and had to be catheterized for relief. Two days later when taking the A.M. vital signs, you note a T-101, P-94, R-18, and BP-124/80. The client tells you he had to go to the bathroom several times during the night and feels tired. You ask if he has any other problems and he tells you his leg feels great, but he did notice that it burned when he urinated this morning. Based upon the above information, you suspect the client has developed a _____ infection of the _____.

7. You are caring for a 67-year-old woman with pneumonia and severe diarrhea. The client has been placed on contact isolation precautions. Upon assessment of her medication history, you discover that the client has a history of upper respiratory infections and has a "stash" of antibiotics at home that she takes when symptoms occur. You recognize this client may be at risk for a nosocomial infection because of _____.

## MULTIPLE CHOICE

Circle the answer that best completes the following statements.

1. Edema to an injured or infected site is which step in the inflammatory response?
   A. vascular
   B. cellular
   C. healing
   D. chemical

2. Nursing interventions for a client with acute inflammation are aimed at which cardinal manifestations of inflammation?
   A. redness, swelling, pain
   B. warmth, pain, impaired function
   C. swelling, impaired function, pain
   D. redness, warmth, impaired function

3. You examine a WBC count ordered for a client. The WBC count is 3,000/mm$^3$. This value most likely indicates:
   A. leukocytosis, a bacterial infection.
   B. leukopenia, a viral infection.
   C. This is a normal WBC count.
   D. No information can be obtained from this value.

4. When interpreting a WBC differential, a "shift to the left" indicates which of the following?
   A. large amount of immature WBCs severe infection.
   B. large amount of mature WBCs severe infection.
   C. large amount of immature WBCs cancer.
   D. large amount of mature WBCs cancer.

5. Cultures of blood, wounds, or other infected body fluids should be obtained:
   A. 30 minutes after the first dose of antimicrobial therapy.
   B. 24 hours after the first dose of antimicrobial therapy.
   C. 24 and 36 hours after the first dose of antimicrobial therapy.
   D. prior to beginning antimicrobial therapy.

6. The nurse wears personal protective equipment (gloves, mask, gown, and goggles) to break which link in the chain of infection?
   A. microorganism
   B. reservoir
   C. portal of exit
   D. portal of entry

7. Choose the nursing intervention that will break the chain of infection in a client with a contagious respiratory infection.
   A. Administer antibiotic therapy.
   B. Have all visitors wear a mask.
   C. Practice meticulous hand washing.
   D. All of the above.

8. Which of the following microorganisms is easily transmitted from client to client on a nurse's hands?
   A. *Escherichia coli*
   B. *Staphylococcus aureus*
   C. streptococci
   D. enterococcus

9. Inappropriate use of antibiotics contributes to nosocomial infections because:
   A. some bacteria survive and become resistant to the antibiotic.
   B. normal flora are killed.
   C. nosocomial infections only occur in those people who are taking antibiotics.
   D. none of the above.

10. You are changing the linens for a client with a draining wound infected with MRSA. Which precautions should be taken?
    A. Wear gloves, gown, and mask to change linens.
    B. Wear gloves to change linens.
    C. Wear gloves and gown to change linens.
    D. No precautions are necessary.

11. Which of the following clients is at the greatest risk of infection?
    A. 42-year-old client with a rib fracture
    B. 56-year-old client with enlarged prostate who drinks cranberry juice
    C. 62-year-old client with a history of TB exposure
    D. 76-year-old client with recent CVA and no flu vaccine

12. Penicillin should be taken:
    A. with food.
    B. with yogurt.
    C. with water.
    D. until symptoms dissipate.

13. An example of a cephalosporin is:
    A. cefazolin.
    B. nafcillin.
    C. potassium clavulanate.
    D. gentamycin.

14. Clients requiring CDC Tier 2 Transmission-based Precautions have:
    A. rare microorganisms transmitted by blood to any host.
    B. virulent microorganisms easily transmittable to any host.
    C. nosocomial infections.
    D. community-acquired infections.

15. You are caring for a hospitalized client who develops chickenpox after a visit from his 5-year-old son. Your client will require which level of precaution?
    A. Negative air pressure room; visitors must wear a mask.
    B. Private room with visitors wearing a mask within 3 feet.
    C. Gown and gloves required if entering room.
    D. No precautions other than standard are necessary.

Read the following situation. Unscramble the words and define each term. Answer the questions using the nursing process of assessment, diagnosis, planning, implementation, and evaluation.

A nursing home resident is being admitted for fever and treatment of a skin tear to the lower leg resulting from a fall. Your assessment reveals: T-99.8, P-92, R-22, BP-128/82. *Malnfmiantoi* is noted at the wound site. *Ytsienhiapmld* is observed. The physician's assessment includes the diagnosis of *leltuciisl,* suspicion of *ksyetsulocio,* and a nosocomial wound infection. The physician orders a CBC, wound culture, antibiotics, and wound care.

1. In addition to the physical assessment, what other information would be important to obtain?
2. Discuss two nursing diagnoses that would be appropriate for this client.
3. What is the most likely antibiotic to be prescribed and what are the nursing implications?
4. Document the wound care in the nursing notes.

# Chapter 11

# Caring for Clients with Altered Immunity

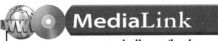

**www.prenhall.com/burke**

Use the address above to access the free, interactive Companion Website created for this textbook. Get hints, instant feedback, and textbook references to chapter-related NCLEX-style questions. Link to other interesting sites.

**Audio Glossary:**

Use the Companion Website, or the CD-ROM disk enclosed with your textbook, to hear the pronunciation of key terms in this chapter.

The immune system is designed to keep foreign substances out of the body and to seek out and destroy these invaders. When the immune system malfunctions, the human body is unable to protect itself. The smallest infection can produce a serious life-threatening situation.

## ANATOMY AND PHYSIOLOGY

Match each term with its appropriate definition.

1. _____ Antigen
2. _____ Allergen
3. _____ Lymphoid system
4. _____ HLA
5. _____ Cell-mediated immunity
6. _____ Humoral immunity
7. _____ Natural immunity
8. _____ Acquired immunity
9. _____ Active immunity
10. _____ Passive immunity

A. Cell surface markers unique to each person
B. B cells produce antibodies
C. Type of antigen responsible for allergic response
D. Artificially received as a result of a vaccination
E. Substance capable of producing an immune response
F. Antibodies received via the placenta
G. Main source of lymphocytes in the body
H. Comprised of helper and killer T cells
I. Memory cells are produced against specific antigens
J. Innate resistance to foreign substances

## FILL IN THE BLANK

Fill in the blanks with the appropriate word or phrase.

1. The nurse is preparing a gamma globulin injection for a client who was exposed to hepatitis B. The type of immunity provided by this injection is called _____.

2. A student tells you that he needs proof of his measles vaccination. Your clinic did not administer the vaccination. You anticipate the physician will order _____.

3. The physician orders a flu vaccination for an elderly client. Prior to giving the injection you must ask about allergies to _____.

4. Insect stings and food allergies produce a type of reaction called _____.

5. An AIDS client complains of a sore mouth. Upon inspection, the nurse observes white patches on the tongue. This condition is known as _____.

6. You are a nurse in an oncology clinic. A client, who received a bone marrow transplant 1 month ago, presents with a rash on his palms and persistent bloody diarrhea. You suspect the client may be developing _____.

7. During the assessment of an HIV patient, the nurse observes reddish-purple lesions on the arms and legs. This form of cancer is called _____.

## MULTIPLE CHOICE

Circle the answer that best completes the following statements.

1. The function of the bone marrow is to
   A. mature lymphocytes into T cells.
   B. filter out damaged RBCs.
   C. manufacture blood cells.
   D. filter out foreign particles.

2. A nursing assistant tells the nurse that a rash is developing on her hands. The most appropriate response should be:
   A. "What are you washing your hands with?"
   B. "Don't wear any gloves when you give a bath."
   C. "Which type of gloves are you using?"
   D. "Do you have an allergy to peanuts?"

3. The nurse is providing teaching for a client scheduled for allergy skin testing. The client asks what kind of preparation is needed for the test. The best response might be:
   A. "You don't need to do anything."
   B. "Oh, I have to gather all the supplies for the doctor."
   C. "Nothing, but epinephrine will be given prior to the test."
   D. None of the above.

4. Adults should have a tetanus toxoid (Td) every:
   A. year.
   B. 2 years.
   C. 5 years.
   D. 10 years.

5. The nurse is teaching a "safe-sex" class at a local high school. He knows that further teaching is necessary when one of the students states:
   A. "As long as I use a condom, I won't get anyone pregnant."
   B. "Wow, I didn't know that condoms should be made of latex."
   C. "I shouldn't have unprotected sex."
   D. "I guess that the condoms in my wallet are too old to use now."

6. You are assessing a client's immune status. Which of the following must be included in the documentation?
   A. recent exposure to a friend with active tuberculosis
   B. hernia repair 4 years ago
   C. diagnosis of post-traumatic syndrome
   D. history of mumps at the age of 6 years

7. You are preparing for the NCLEX-PN® by reviewing your immunology notes. Which of the following is not considered a part of the immune system?
   A. thymus gland
   B. appendix
   C. gallbladder
   D. spleen

8. A client has been taking diphenhydramine for hay fever symptoms. Which of the following is not a common side effect of the medication?
   A. drowsiness
   B. sedation
   C. urinary retention
   D. thirst

9. A client is taking cyclosporin to prevent rejection of his new kidney. The daily lab work is faxed to your unit. Which of the following would require a call to the physician?
   A. glucose 93
   B. BUN 10
   C. WBC 3000
   D. platelet count 150,000

10. You feel confident that your client, an organ transplant recipient, understands your discharge instructions when he says:
    A. "I'm going to take my temperature and weight at the same time every day."
    B. "I will take my Cellcept at the first sign of a fever."
    C. "As long as I don't drink after my children when they are sick, I am safe from infection."
    D. "I won't have to see my doctor unless I don't feel well."

11. Nursing care for any immunocompromised client includes removing invasive lines as soon as possible. The rationale for this intervention is that:
    A. the client can go home sooner.
    B. fewer sites are available for bacterial invasion.
    C. the client is more comfortable.
    D. signs of infection are easier to monitor.

12. Isolation precautions for the transplant client are designed to:
    A. reduce possible microorganisms transferred by the client.
    B. reduce possible microorganisms transferred to the client.
    C. reduce the risk of rejection.
    D. all of the above.

13. Your patient, a 62-year-old female, has recently been diagnosed with rheumatoid arthritis. She tells you that she just doesn't feel like getting up in the mornings. Her housework is not getting done. An appropriate nursing diagnosis might be:
    A. Disturbed Body Image
    B. Fatigue
    C. Ineffective Individual Coping
    D. Acute Pain

14. In addition to the ELISA, which of the following tests is used to diagnose HIV?
    A. HIV viral load
    B. CD4 cell count
    C. Western blot
    D. all of the above

15. The appropriate statement to a client who admitted to "sharing a needle" should be:
    A. "If your HIV test is negative after three months, you have nothing to fear."
    B. "Don't worry, the HIV virus is only transmitted in semen."
    C. "Seroconversion usually occurs in six to twenty-four weeks."
    D. "Try not to think about it."

## CRITICAL THINKING EXERCISE

Read the following situation. Unscramble the words and define each term. Answer the questions using the nursing process of assessment, diagnosis, planning, implementation, and evaluation.

A 42-year-old female has been admitted to your floor with a primary diagnosis of *DISA*. The client sought emergency care for unrelenting diarrhea and malaise. She tells you that she has lost 25 pounds during the last 3 months. The secondary medical diagnosis for this client is wasting syndrome. The history reveals *ndidiaissnac* and *lmyomahp*. She mentions that she had recently been treated for cervical *plasiadys* on an outpatient basis. She begins to cry. "I just don't think I can handle this anymore."

1. In addition to the physical assessment, what other information would be important to obtain?
2. Discuss two nursing diagnoses that would be appropriate for this client.
3. What nursing interventions might be initiated in response to the client's statement?
4. Make an entry into the client's medical record using the SOAP format (subjective, objective, assessment, planning).

# Chapter 12

## Caring for Clients with Cancer

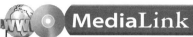

**MediaLink**

**www.prenhall.com/burke**

Use the address above to access the free, interactive Companion Website created for this textbook. Get hints, instant feedback, and textbook references to chapter-related NCLEX-style questions. Link to other interesting sites.

**Audio Glossary:**

Use the Companion Website, or the CD-ROM disk enclosed with your textbook, to hear the pronunciation of key terms in this chapter.

Cancer is characterized by abnormal, unrestricted cell proliferation. Malignant tumors invade healthy tissues and compete with normal cells for oxygen, nutrients, and physical space. The reactions of clients depend on the particular diagnosis, location, stage, treatment modalities, effects on bodily functions, and prognosis.

## CANCER TERMINOLOGY

Match each term with its appropriate definition.

1. _____ Cancer
2. _____ Oncologist
3. _____ Neoplasm
4. _____ Metastasis
5. _____ Oncogenes
6. _____ Lymphocytes
7. _____ Anorexia-cachexia syndrome
8. _____ Classification
9. _____ Computed tomography
10. _____ Tumor markers

A. Process of invading other tissues
B. White blood cells
C. Converts normal cells into cancer cells
D. Cancer specialist
E. Group of neoplastic diseases
F. Effect of cancer cells on metabolism
G. Any new abnormal growth
H. Imaging technique
I. Biochemical indicator of malignancy
J. Naming of tumor tissue or cell of origin

## FILL IN THE BLANK

Fill in the blanks with the appropriate word or phrase.

1. Within the nucleus of normal cells, chromosomes containing _____ molecules carry the genetic information that controls the synthesis of proteins.

2. _____ refers to the relative size of the tumor and extent of the disease.

3. The leading type of cancer in the United States is _____.

4. It is well documented that long-term exposure to secondhand smoke increases the risk for _____ and _____ cancers.

5. The recreational drug that has been linked to chromosome damage is _____.

6. _____ disrupts the cell cycle in various phases by disturbing normal cell metabolism and replication.

7. The community program that has allowed many cancer patients to spend their last days at home is called _____.

## MULTIPLE CHOICE

Circle the answer that best completes the following statements.

1. Nurses are aware that the second-leading cause of death in people over the age of 65 is:
   A. chronic obstructive pulmonary disease.
   B. end-stage renal failure.
   C. cancer.
   D. coronary artery disease.

2. You are teaching a health class at a local retirement center. When discussing the potential for prostate cancer in the older male, you include the following teaching point:
   A. Prostate self-examination every week.
   B. X-ray of the prostate gland after the age of 65.
   C. Screening for the presence of PSA.
   D. CT scan of the chest to rule out metastasis.

3. Mrs. Jackson has been diagnosed with breast cancer and metastasis to the spinal cord. She is paralyzed from the waist down and requires assistance with ADLs. Which of the following nursing diagnoses would be the most appropriate at this time?
   A. Risk for Infection
   B. Risk for Impaired Skin Integrity
   C. Risk for Injury
   D. Risk for Caregiver Role Strain

4. A divorced mother of four school-aged children is hospitalized with inoperable brain cancer. The client voices concern over the care for her children after her death. The best response should be:
   A. "You are going to live for a while longer and will have time to make arrangements."
   B. "Won't your ex-husband care for his kids after your death?"
   C. "I wouldn't worry about that right now. Just focus on getting well."
   D. "Would you like to share your thoughts with me?"

5. Interleukin-2 is used as therapy for a client with metastatic renal cancer. The nurse recognizes that the goal of this type of treatment might be:
   A. selectively altering the DNA of malignant cells.
   B. enhancing the client's immunologic response to tumor cells.
   C. stimulating malignant cells to enter mitosis.
   D. preventing bone marrow depression.

6. After the implantation of a radioactive cervical implant in an outpatient clinic, it is important to teach the client to:
   A. avoid close contact with others.
   B. limit activity to 30 minutes per day.
   C. eat three nutritious meals every day.
   D. dispose of the implant in the trash if it becomes dislodged.

7. You are reviewing a client's history prior to assisting in the development of a nursing care plan. You note that the patient has been diagnosed with colon carcinoma. The staging classification is $T_{IS}$. You understand that this represents:
   A. a tumor with no metastasis.
   B. no evidence of a primary tumor.
   C. a tumor that is localized and encapsulated.
   D. no abnormal lymph nodes.

8. The American Cancer Society has outlined several cancer warning signals. If all of the following are true, which signal would be particularly important to the chronic smoker?
   A. obvious change in mole or wart
   B. a sore that does not heal
   C. nagging cough
   D. change in bowel habit

9. The nurse has completed a physical assessment on a patient diagnosed with pancreatic cancer. Which of these findings indicate poor nutritional status?
   A. positive muscle tone
   B. good skin turgor
   C. moist oral membranes
   D. distended abdomen

10. A gastric cancer client is receiving high doses of 5-FU. Based on your knowledge of the side effects of this chemotherapy drug, which nursing intervention should take priority in the client's care?
    A. six small meals a day
    B. increase PO fluids
    C. assess lungs for coarse rales
    D. monitor lab values for the presence of uric acid

11. The drug tamoxifen is generally used in the treatment of:
    A. breast cancer.
    B. prostate cancer.
    C. small-cell lung cancer.
    D. bladder cancer.

12. A client who is being treated on an outpatient basis for kidney cancer telephones the nurse on duty and states, "I just don't think I can take any more treatments." The best response of the nurse should be:
    A. "Okay, I'll let your doctor know right away."
    B. "You sound terrible, what's the matter?"
    C. "Would you like to talk about your concerns?"
    D. "Please tell me your concerns."

13. Which of the following are not characteristics of a malignant neoplasm?
    A. rapid growth
    B. well-defined borders
    C. noncohesive
    D. invasive

14. The nurse is teaching the client about the care of radiation skin markings. Of the following, which should be most emphasized during the session?
    A. Protect the skin from sunlight.
    B. Do not wash off the markings.
    C. Do not apply heat or cold to the marked areas.
    D. Wear loose clothing.

15. The tool of choice for diagnosing head and neck cancer is:
    A. MRI.
    B. CT scan.
    C. x-ray imaging.
    D. ultrasonography.

## CRITICAL THINKING EXERCISE

Read the following situation. Unscramble the words and define each term. Answer the questions using the nursing process of assessment, diagnosis, planning, implementation, and evaluation.

A 64-year-old female was admitted to the oncology unit for treatment of advanced breast *ccearn*. Her history is as follows: *gingast iiialcssfcaton* $T_4N_{3b}M_3$, fracture of right hip 5 months ago, *nnnnctiioet* of urine times 3 weeks, severe back pain. The physician has ordered *lavNodex* as the preferred treatment of choice. The physical exam reveals anorexia-cachexia. The client's vital signs are T-100.0, P-96, R-14, BP-148/90.

1. Interpret the staging classification for this patient.
2. Name two nursing diagnoses that would be appropriate at this time.
3. List two interventions for each diagnosis.
4. How would the nurse document the anorexia-cachexia syndrome in the nursing notes?

# Chapter 13

## Caring for Clients Experiencing Shock, Trauma, or Critical Illness

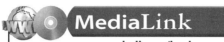

**MediaLink**

www.prenhall.com/burke

Use the address above to access the free, interactive Companion Website created for this textbook. Get hints, instant feedback, and textbook references to chapter-related NCLEX-style questions. Link to other interesting sites.

**Audio Glossary:**

Use the Companion Website, or the CD-ROM disk enclosed with your textbook, to hear the pronunciation of key terms in this chapter.

Shock is a life-threatening event that can take place in minutes or over several days. The nurse must be able to observe and correlate subtle signs that may develop from trauma or critical illnesses in order to provide clients with effective nursing care.

## SHOCK AND TRAUMA TERMINOLOGY

Match each term with its appropriate definition.

1. _____ Triage
2. _____ Shunt
3. _____ Shock
4. _____ Contusion

5. _____ Acuity
6. _____ ARDS
7. _____ Antigen
8. _____ Hypoxia
9. _____ Mottling

10. _____ Laceration

A. Discoloration of the skin
B. Diminished oxygenation to the tissues
C. Irregular skin tear
D. Classification system used to determine illness level
E. Complete respiratory failure
F. Foreign substance
G. Injury to tissue without skin breakage
H. System to identify priority care
I. Movement of fluids from one area to another
J. Peripheral circulatory failure

## FILL IN THE BLANK

Fill in the blanks with the appropriate word or phrase.

1. A client arrives at the emergency room with a partially severed arm. His friend states, "Jack must have lost at least a quart of blood." Assessment reveals cool, moist skin with a capillary refill of >5 seconds. Vital signs: T-96, P-142 weak and regular, R-36 shallow, BP-90/40. You anticipate that Jack is in _____.

2. Mrs. Wilson, injured in a motor vehicle crash, states that she believes her chest hit the steering wheel. An hour after your initial assessment, Mrs. Wilson complains of SOB. You discover an absence of left breath sounds. You suspect the client is experiencing _____.

3. Alex has sustained second- and third-degree burns over 50% of his body. He continues to lose large amounts of serous fluid. Based on your knowledge of burns, you believe that Alex will develop _____.

4. A young child is brought into the clinic in respiratory distress. His mother tells you that he was bitten by a hornet. The physician will probably make a diagnosis of _____.

5. Mr. Elphonso is admitted to the hospital with a fever of 103.6°F, P-110, R-32, and BP-110/50. His wife tells you that he was seen in the clinic 10 days ago for an infected cut. Urine and blood cultures indicate 4+ bacteria. Based on these findings, you believe that this client may be diagnosed with _____.

6. Adam has been in a motorcycle crash and a piece of debris is embedded in his thigh. This type of injury is classified as _____ trauma.

7. A 17-year-old male has been brought into the emergency room after being beaten by a fellow classmate. He has multiple injuries, including a lacerated spleen and ruptured bowel. In addition to a risk of hemorrhage, this client is also at risk for the development of _____.

## MULTIPLE CHOICE

Circle the answer that best completes the following statements.

1. Which of the following would not be considered the cause of a blood pressure drop in the condition known as shock?
   A. loss of blood volume
   B. severe histamine reaction
   C. decreased cardiac output
   D. low HGB and HCT

2. A patient with end-stage kidney disease is at risk for the progressive stage of shock because:
   A. the kidneys are not able to concentrate urine.
   B. the renin-angiotensin system is not functioning properly.
   C. the kidneys are not able to metabolize toxins.
   D. the patient is not at risk for this stage of shock.

3. Mr. Jones admits to the emergency room in shock after a motor vehicle crash. He is disoriented and unable to follow simple commands. You know that this is due to:
   A. decreased blood flow to the brain.
   B. vasoconstriction of the great vessels.
   C. shunting of blood to the GI tract.
   D. the stress caused by the crash.

4. A person is most likely to experience an anaphylactic reaction:
   A. within 5 minutes of exposure to the allergen.
   B. after the second day of exposure to an allergen.
   C. when exposed to any allergen that produces hypersensitivity.
   D. during the second exposure to the allergen.

5. Mrs. James is recovering from septic shock. She has extensive tissue damage to her liver and kidneys due to:
   A. bacterial infection.
   B. reaction to the antibiotic.
   C. endotoxins released into the bloodstream.
   D. microemboli.

6. The administration of oxygen is an appropriate therapy for all types of shock because:
   A. oxygen eases the respiratory effort.
   B. lack of oxygen is the primary cause of tissue damage.
   C. oxygen is considered a comforting measure.
   D. lack of oxygen increases the risk for mental confusion.

7. A patient with B negative blood requires an emergency transfusion of whole blood. You know that in order to be compatible, the blood obtained from the lab must be:
   A. O negative or B negative.
   B. O positive or B negative or B positive.
   C. B negative or AB negative.
   D. B positive or B negative.

8. The goal of epinephrine therapy is to:
   A. promote bronchiole dilatation and increase arterial BP.
   B. reverse the histamine effects.
   C. prevent a delayed reaction to an antigen.
   D. prevent a delayed reaction to an antibody.

9. If there is blood loss or systemic vasodilatation, you will expect the doctor to order:
   A. oxygen.
   B. alpha-adrenergic medication.
   C. beta-adrenergic medication.
   D. cardiotonics.

10. Mr. Bruce has a nursing diagnosis of Ineffective Tissue Perfusion related to cardiopulmonary failure. Your primary nursing intervention will be to:
    A. maintain airway and blood oxygen saturation.
    B. check vital signs every hour.
    C. obtain daily weights.
    D. assess bowel function every shift.

11. A client has been in the trauma room for 15 hours after experiencing a severe injury to her back. You suspect that the shock of the accident is resolving because:
    A. she stops asking where she is.
    B. her urine output has increased to 40 mL/hr and the pedal pulses are palpable.
    C. oxygen saturation levels have been >94% for the last 60 minutes.
    D. her blood pressure is stable at 100/50.

12. You are pulled to the emergency room to assist with a sudden influx of patients. When you arrive, the charge nurse says to "pick a patient." Who will you see first?
    A. 50-year-old, chest pain, BP-140/80
    B. 26-year-old chronic asthmatic, R-30, $O_2$ saturation-92% room air, BP-120/72
    C. 18-year-old, leg trauma from a MVA, controlled hemorrhage, BP-139/80
    D. 42-year-old, fall from roof, slurred speech, BP-80/40, P-160, R-36 shallow

13. The home health nurse is visiting 92-year-old Mr. Smith, who has been diagnosed with Parkinson's disease and early macular degeneration. Mr. Smith is at risk for trauma related to weakness and poor eyesight. Which of the following would decrease the fall potential for this patient?
    A. Review the medications with the doctor.
    B. Assist the patient to rearrange the furniture.
    C. Increase the number of lamps in the house.
    D. Encourage him to move into assisted-living housing.

14. Andrea has been diagnosed with an allergy to peanuts. You are providing nutritional education. You know that she needs further teaching when she says:
    A. "I need to ask what type of oil is used to fry the foods."
    B. "I need to read all food labels very carefully."
    C. "If I can't see the nuts, then I can eat the food."
    D. "I need to keep Benadryl with me at all times."

15. The school nurse is providing first-aid training to a group of high school athletic students. When she discusses hemorrhaging, she remembers to include:
    A. apply a tourniquet immediately to bleeding limbs.
    B. call for help, then apply a tourniquet.
    C. always move an injured person with the head lower than the feet.
    D. check for immediate danger, call for help, apply pressure.

## CRITICAL THINKING EXERCISE

Read the following situation. Unscramble the words and define each term. Answer the questions using the nursing process of assessment, diagnosis, planning, implementation, and evaluation.

Mr. Jenkins is a 76-year-old male admitted to the surgical floor after an ORIF of the left hip. His vital signs are T-97.8, P-80, R-18, BP-138/68. Darvocet N100 tab, 2 PO q 4–6 hours prn, is ordered for pain. His condition is stable. Dressing is dry and intact. Pedal pulses are strong. You return to the unit after being off for 2 days and discover that Mr. Jenkins has been complaining constantly about pain; otherwise he is fine. After report, you find that his vital signs are T-101, P-116, R-26, BP-110/60. He is alert and very *xiousan*. His skin is flushed and damp. You note that his *aldep suples* are weak. The dressing on his hip has not been changed for several days. When you expose the wound, four staples appear loose and there is significant bloody drainage from the site. His *utputo rineu* is 375 mL/12 hours. Based on this information, you suspect that Mr. Jenkins has developed *sceipt choks*.

1.  What effect did the frequent Darvocet doses have on Mr. Jenkin's temperature?
2.  What factors contributed to the development of sepsis?
3.  When you call the doctor, what information should you report?
4.  Would the issue of poor nursing care be presented in Mr. Jenkin's chart? Explain.

# Chapter 14

## Loss, Grief, and End-of-Life Care

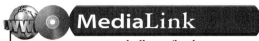

All clients experience loss, grief, and death in a personal manner. An understanding of the grieving process brings awareness and the ability to develop effective interventions for terminally ill clients and their families.

## ANATOMY OF LOSS, GRIEF, AND DEATH

Match each term with its appropriate definition.

1. _____ Loss
2. _____ Grief
3. _____ Death
4. _____ Advanced directives
5. _____ Durable power of attorney
6. _____ Living will
7. _____ Comfort measures
8. _____ Involuntary euthanasia
9. _____ Hospice
10. _____ DNR

A. Irreversible cessation of brain function
B. Personal expression of life-saving interventions
C. Planning for future health care/financial matters
D. Providing only soothing interventions
E. Emotional response to loss
F. Mercy killing
G. Giving power to another for decisions in care
H. Amount of diminished quantity
I. Provider of end-of-life care
J. Do not restore to life

## FILL IN THE BLANK

Fill in the blanks with the appropriate word or phrase.

1. The stage of experiencing loss begins with a defensive statement known as _____.

2. When a person enters the stage of realization about an impending loss, the initial reaction is _____.

3. The core of human existence, integrating and transcending the physical, emotional, intellectual, and social dimensions, is called _____.

4. A document that states each person has the right to be cared for by sensitive and knowledgeable people is known as the _____.

5. Specific terms for developing and providing information and counseling about advanced directives may be found in the law known as the _____.

6. The Greek word for a painless, easy, or good death is _____.

7. The combined knowledge and skills of the health care team are known as _____ care.

## MULTIPLE CHOICE

Circle the answer that best completes the following statements.

1. A nursing student tells the nurse that she has heard the "death rattle" while caring for a client. The best explanation of this term is:
   A. creaking of the joints.
   B. gurgling of fluids in the lungs and throat.
   C. air bubbles in the stomach.
   D. teeth grinding.

2. Factors that may interfere with successful grieving include all of the following except:
   A. traumatic circumstances surrounding the loss.
   B. perceived inability to share the loss.
   C. lack of social recognition of the loss.
   D. mutual understanding and relationships.

3. The process of viewing the body after death best supports which of the following statements?
   A. Provides the resolution of the death experience for most families.
   B. Increases anxiety levels.
   C. Allows family members an avenue of escape from the truth.
   D. Supports the family members' decision for a DNR.

4. Which of the following would most likely interfere with the nurse–client relationship during the final stages of impending death?
   A. unresolved issues of the nurse's perception of death
   B. anger with the physician for writing a DNR order
   C. inability to notify the client's family of the impending death
   D. personal knowledge of the client's family situation

5. A nurse is caring for an elderly Chinese-American and notices that a piece of handkerchief is lying on her chest. The nurse should immediately:
   A. throw the cloth in the trashcan.
   B. place the item on the bedside table.
   C. speak to the family about the significance of the gesture.
   D. ignore the distraction.

6. An American Indian family appears to be throwing a party in the room where their grandmother is dying. Your best response would be to:
   A. remind the family of the seriousness of the situation.
   B. join in the festivities.
   C. acknowledge the cultural tradition.
   D. report the incident to the nursing supervisor.

7. A nursing assistant refuses to care for a dying person. The most appropriate response by the nurse would be:
   A. "Okay, I'll reassign you to another patient."
   B. "Please tell me what concerns you about this patient's care."
   C. "Grow up, death is a part of life!"
   D. "Just get someone else to do this assignment for you."

8. Physical and emotional care is important to the dying person. Which of the following interventions would be the most comforting during the last stages of life?
   A. Change the linens every 2 hours.
   B. Provide frequent oral care.
   C. Encourage a family member to spend time at the bedside.
   D. Tell the client that everything will be okay.

9. The concern that most clients voice as they near the end of their lives is:
   A. the fear of dying alone.
   B. the fear of pain.
   C. the fear of leaving family members.
   D. the fear of bodily function loss.

10. You are helping another nurse to turn a comatose, dying client. The nurse states, "Whew, this lady sure is fat." Your best response should be:
    A. "That's not a nice thing to say."
    B. "Yeah, you got that right!"
    C. "Let's talk outside after we are finished."
    D. Say nothing, just glare at the nurse.

11. A 94-year-old client refuses to eat breakfast. According to the shift report, she has not eaten in 3 days. Your next action should be to:
    A. keep trying to feed her by placing the food in her mouth.
    B. read the physician's notes in her chart.
    C. call the family and ask them to bring food from home.
    D. start an IV of $D_5W$ to provide calories.

12. Your patient, diagnosed with inoperable stomach cancer, wants to die at home. He asks you what organization might help him die peacefully. Which of the following would be the most appropriate community referral resource?
    A. Meals-on-Wheels
    B. community mental health centers
    C. Hospice of America
    D. American Association of Colleges of Nursing

13. The nurse is aware that a terminal patient has stopped breathing, and responds to the call only after drinking a cup of coffee. This type of behavior is considered:
    A. routine in most facilities.
    B. malpractice if the patient has not been designated a DNR.
    C. unprofessional and inhumane.
    D. appropriate considering the patient's prognosis.

14. You are caring for a patient with end-stage renal disease. The patient is fully alert and competent. The husband asks you to "give my wife just a little more pain medication to completely stop her from suffering." Your best response would be to:
    A. clarify the request.
    B. privately administer more medication.
    C. speak to the wife about her pain level.
    D. call the physician and report the incident.

15. You overhear a patient state, "If you make me well, God, I will try to be a better person." You know that this type of statement is one of the stages of the grieving process known as:
    A. anger.
    B. bargaining.
    C. denial.
    D. depression.

## CRITICAL THINKING EXERCISE

Read the following situation. Unscramble the words and define each term. Answer the questions using the nursing process of assessment, diagnosis, planning, implementation, and evaluation.

Mrs. Gash, age 55, has a history of colon-rectal cancer with *satsisatme* to the liver. She has been hospitalized three times within the last year. Her doctor referred the family to a *ciespho* program for the duration of her care. Mr. Gash has accepted his wife's prognosis but acknowledges that Mrs. Gash has become depressed and angry during the last several weeks. As Mrs. Gash's pain increases, her cooperation with the hospice nurse has diminished. The family is concerned that Mrs. Gash has not discussed the need for any *vanedcda viescedrit, vinlig llswi,* or DNR considerations. Any attempt to bring up the subject results in increased anxiety and frustration for all family members.

1. What is the most important concern for Mrs. Gash at the present time?
2. How should the hospice nurse address the issue of Mrs. Gash's uncooperative behavior?
3. What nursing diagnosis might be recommended for Mr. Gash?
4. Which items discussed must be documented in the nursing notes?

# Chapter 15

## The Endocrine System and Assessment

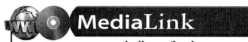

**www.prenhall.com/burke**

Use the address above to access the free, interactive Companion Website created for this textbook. Get hints, instant feedback, and textbook references to chapter-related NCLEX-style questions. Link to other interesting sites.

**Audio Glossary:**

Use the Companion Website, or the CD-ROM disk enclosed with your textbook, to hear the pronunciation of key terms in this chapter.

The endocrine system is composed of seven glands that serve to regulate the internal environment of the human body. Each gland releases specific hormones in response to the needs of the client.

## ANATOMY AND PHYSIOLOGY

Match each term with its appropriate definition.

1. __D__ Pancreas
2. __E__ Hypothalamus
3. __B__ Pituitary
4. __G__ Adrenal cortex
5. __A__ Iodine
6. __F__ Islets of Langerhans
7. __H__ Epinephrine
8. __C__ Parathyroid
9. __J__ Thyroid
10. __I__ Adrenal medulla

A. Necessary for proper functioning of the thyroid

B. Master gland

C. Increases calcium blood levels

D. Secretes digestive enzymes and releases insulin and glucagon into the bloodstream

E. Regulates temperature, fluid volume, and growth

F. Produces insulin

G. Produces corticosteroids

H. A counterregulatory hormone

I. Produces hormones known as catecholamines

J. Reduces excess calcium in the blood

## FILL IN THE BLANK

Fill in the blanks with the appropriate word or phrase.

1. A client comes to the clinic complaining of <u>polyuria</u>, <u>extreme thirst</u>, and <u>fatigue</u>. Your assessment findings indicate tachycardia and signs of dehydration. You suspect this client will be diagnosed with ___diabetes insipidus___ .

2. The nurse is assessing a male client and notices an enlargement in breast tissue. This condition is called ___gynecomastia___

3. A classic sign of an overactive thyroid condition in which the eyeballs appear to bulge from the sockets is referred to as ___exophthalmos___.

4. The most common endocrine disorders in older adults include thyroid abnormalities and an increased risk for ___DM___ .

5. A client is concerned about the swelling in her neck. There is a visible mass in the thyroid region. The nurse anticipates that the doctor will explain to the client that she has a ___goiter___ .

6. Hormone secretion is triggered by some stimulus, internal or external to the body. The rising levels of hormones, in turn, prevent the continuous release of additional hormones. This delicate balance cycle is referred to as ___negative feedback___

## MULTIPLE CHOICE

Circle the answer that best completes the following statements.

1. A patient, diagnosed with diabetes, tells you that he is having increased blood sugars 2 hours after meals. Based on this statement, the nurse prepares a care plan for a nursing diagnosis of:
   A. Disturbed Body Image related to physical changes.
   B. Activity Intolerance related to increased blood sugars.
   C. Pain related to increased abdominal girth after meals.
   D. Deficient Knowledge related to diagnosis of diabetes.

2. An elderly patient is taking a diuretic for mild congestive heart failure. He has recently been admitted to the hospital for SIADH. Which of the following nursing interventions must be included in the plan of care?
   A. Provide oral mouth care at frequent intervals.
   B. Push fluids as tolerated.
   C. Initiate seizure precautions.
   D. Assess respiratory status every 4 hours.

3. Mrs. Leopold presents with a temperature of 99°F, malaise, and says, "I feel tired all the time." Subsequent labs reveal a $T_4$ of 0.5 mcg/dL. You suspect that Mrs. Leopold will be diagnosed with:
   A. Cushing's syndrome.
   B. severe bronchitis.
   C. hypothyroidism.
   D. sepsis.

4. In the medication instructions for a client taking a corticosteroid, you must include which of the following?
   A. Take the medication on an empty stomach.
   B. Do not stop taking the medication without consulting the physician.
   C. Eat foods that are low in potassium.
   D. Maintain a healthy diet.

5. A common GI complaint for a client diagnosed with hypothyroidism is:
   A. frequent stomach pains.
   B. constipation.
   C. bloody stools.
   D. increased peristalsis.

6. A client complains of an "extreme case of the jitters" and a sensation of thumps in her chest. Her lab values indicate an increased level of $T_3$ and $T_4$. Based on this information, the most likely diagnosis will be:
   A. thyrotoxicosis.
   B. cretinism.
   C. hyperparathyroidism.
   D. Cushing's syndrome.

7. A patient, diagnosed with diabetes insipidus, is experiencing tachycardia, poor skin turgor, and a dry mouth. The nurse anticipates the development of a care plan for:
   A. nocturia.
   B. polyuria.
   C. dehydration.
   D. hypernatremia.

8. Mrs. Randall comes to the clinic complaining of a wound on her arm that will not heal. During her assessment, she also admits to some difficulty in concentrating, recent weight gain, and fatigue. Your next question is regarding her urine output, because you suspect:
   A. hyperthyroidism.
   B. hypothyroidism.
   C. Cushing's syndrome.
   D. Addison's disease.

9. A client who has recently developed exophthalmos tells you that she has stopped dating. She tells you that she thought her eyes would return to "normal" after her diagnosis of Graves' disease. A primary nursing diagnosis would be:
   A. Ineffective Health Maintenance
   B. Disturbed Personal Identity
   C. Deficient Knowledge.
   D. Risk for Situational Low Self-Esteem

10. A patient diagnosed with hypoparathyroidism may experience continuous muscle spasms known as:
   A. tetany.
   B. Trousseau.
   C. Chvostek.
   D. tetanic.

## CRITICAL THINKING EXERCISE

Read the following situation. Unscramble the words and define each term. Answer the questions using the nursing process of assessment, diagnosis, planning, implementation, and evaluation.

Mrs. Thompson, 52 years old, is suffering from a type of *xisiscooootrhty* called Graves' disease. After several years of the disease she begins to develop *moothsaxlep*. The doctor has placed her on *zaplotea* with the expectation that when she achieves an euthroid state she will be scheduled for a *sattublo tocythdeiomyr*. You are asked to prepare a teaching plan relating to her surgery.

1. Name two postoperative complications for this type of surgery.
2. List three nursing interventions for each complication.
3. Discuss the rationale for removing a portion of the thyroid gland.
4. What preoperative teaching instructions should be documented in the chart?

# Chapter 16

## Caring for Clients with Endocrine Disorders

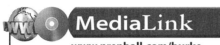
**MediaLink**
www.prenhall.com/burke

Use the address above to access the free, interactive Companion Website created for this textbook. Get hints, instant feedback, and textbook references to chapter-related NCLEX-style questions. Link to other interesting sites.

**Audio Glossary:**

Use the Companion Website, or the CD-ROM disk enclosed with your textbook, to hear the pronunciation of key terms in this chapter.

When the delicate balance of the hormone levels is disturbed, the client experiences a vast array of symptoms that directly affect homeostasis.

## ANATOMY AND PHYSIOLOGY

Match each term with its appropriate definition.

1. __D__ SIADH
2. __E__ Dwarfism
3. __B__ Pituitary adenoma
4. __G__ Hyperthyroidism
5. __A__ Diabetes insipidus
6. __F__ Graves' disease
7. __A__ Addison's disease
8. __C__ Osmolarity
9. __J__ Tetany
10. __I__ Thyroiditis

A. Results from antidiuretic hormone insufficiency
B. Stimulates the hypersecretion of growth hormone that causes acromegaly
C. Concentration of particles in the blood
D. Caused by an excess production of antidiuretic hormone
E. Caused by inadequate production of growth hormone
F. Hyperthyroidism
G. Excessive production of thyroid hormone
H. Insufficient amounts of adrenal cortex hormones
I. Common cause of primary hypothyroidism
J. Occurs with reduced calcium in the blood

## FILL IN THE BLANK

Fill in the blanks with the appropriate word or phrase.

1. Tommy, a 20-year-old, has had a thyroidectomy. Two days after his surgery, Tommy is still unable to speak above a whisper. You anticipate the physician will document _laryngeal nerve damage_.

2. While helping a client to the bathroom, you observe that he has an unusually enlarged forehead, protruding jaw, and wears a size 12 shoe. Based on your knowledge of endocrine disorders, you suspect this client has been diagnosed with _acromegaly_.

3. An abnormal condition created by the overproduction of the growth hormone is called _gigantism_.

4. A life-threatening form of hypothyroidism that occurs in winter months is known as _myxedema coma_.

5. Hashimoto's thyroiditis is classified as a(n) _autoimmune_ because antibodies destroy thyroid tissue. _disorder_

## MULTIPLE CHOICE

Circle the answer that best completes the following statements.

1. A patient, diagnosed with acromegaly, tells you that he is having increased difficulty walking up the stairs at his house. Based on this statement, the nurse prepares a care plan for a nursing diagnosis of:
   A. Disturbed Body Image related to physical changes.
   B. Activity Intolerance related to joint pain.
   C. Pain related to increased weight on joints.
   D. Risk for Injury.

2. Mrs. Kay presents with a temperature of 101°F, malaise, and decreased lung sounds. She has a prescription for L-thyroxine, but tells you that she cannot afford the medication. During the assessment, she rapidly progresses to confusion and subsequently becomes unresponsive. You suspect that Mrs. Kay will be diagnosed with:
   A. thyroiditis.
   B. severe bronchitis.
   C. myxedema.
   D. sepsis.

3. A patient with a blood pressure of 210/160, severe headaches, diaphoresis, tachycardia, and flushed skin is most likely suffering from:
   A. thyroid crisis.
   B. pheochromocytoma.
   C. goiter.
   D. Cushing's syndrome.

4. The nursing intervention that has the highest priority for the patient who has undergone a subtotal thyroidectomy should be:
   A. assess for hemorrhage.
   B. assess for absent bowel sounds.
   C. assess for calcium deficiency.
   D. assess for laryngeal nerve damage.

5. An elderly woman with hyperparathyroidism is also likely to have:
   A. hypophosphatemia.
   B. hyponatremia.
   C. hypercalcemia.
   D. osteomyelitis.

6. The first priority for treating hypoparathyroidism is to administer:
   A. 500 mL of normal saline.
   B. calcium gluconate.
   C. vitamin D.
   D. calciferol.

7. Treatment for the patient with hypothyroidism is:
   A. 500 mL of normal saline.
   B. lifelong.
   C. vitamin D.
   D. short term.

8. Mr. Tracy was diagnosed with hyperthyroidism 15 years ago. Recently he has been experiencing difficulty breathing and swallowing. You suspect:
   A. thyroid cancer.
   B. hyperparathyroidism.
   C. hypocalcemia.
   D. stroke.

9. Mrs. Kim has been complaining of lower back pain for 6 months. Today her labs show elevated levels of serum calcium, PTH, and alkaline phosphatase. These manifestations confirm a diagnosis of:
   A. stroke.
   B. hypocalcemia.
   C. hyperparathyroidism.
   D. thyroid cancer.

10. Nursing care of the client with hypoparathyroidism must consider the client's risk for injury due to:
    A. falls.
    B. tetany.
    C. altered thought processes.
    D. impaired memory.

## CRITICAL THINKING EXERCISE

Read the following situation. Unscramble the words and define each term. Answer the questions using the nursing process of assessment, diagnosis, planning, implementation, and evaluation.

Mrs. Jones, 65 years old, is brought into the emergency room. She presents with *izesseru, dcdiraabyra,* and *pyhoerthiam.* Based on these findings you know she is suffering from a type of *xisiscooootrhty* called myxedema coma. This is a medical *mgeencyer.*

1. Name three causes that may bring about a myxedema coma.
2. List three nursing interventions for each cause.
3. Discuss treatment options and rationales.

# Chapter 17

## Caring for Clients with Diabetes Mellitus

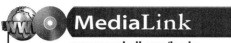

**MediaLink**

**www.prenhall.com/burke**

Use the address above to access the free, interactive Companion Website created for this textbook. Get hints, instant feedback, and textbook references to chapter-related NCLEX-style questions. Link to other interesting sites.

**Audio Glossary:**

Use the Companion Website, or the CD-ROM disk enclosed with your textbook, to hear the pronunciation of key terms in this chapter.

Diabetes is a general term used to describe a group of disorders characterized by excessive urination. Diabetes mellitus specifically refers to problems in the production and/or the utilization of glucose. The client is susceptible to numerous complications, many of which are life-threatening. Compliance with medical treatment is imperative to slow the progress of the illness.

## DIABETES MELLITUS

Match each term with its appropriate definition.

1. _F_ Hyperglycemia
2. _H_ Type 1
3. _G_ Polydipsia
4. _I_ Gangrene
5. _J_ Gluconeogenesis
6. _G_ Ketosis
7. _D_ Distal paresthesia
8. _B_ Insulin
9. _C_ Somogyi effect
10. _A_ Type 2

A. Insufficient insulin production
B. Regulates blood glucose levels
C. Morning rise of blood glucose after low levels at night
D. Numbness or tingling in feet and hands
E. Increased thirst
F. High levels of circulating blood sugar
G. Toxic accumulation of ketone bodies
H. Requires insulin injections to sustain life
I. Necrosis of tissue followed by infection
J. Synthesis of glucose in the liver and kidneys

## FILL IN THE BLANK

Fill in the blanks with the appropriate word or phrase.

1.  The organ that produces digestive enzymes and regulates the amount of glucose in the blood is called the _pancreas_.

2. In response to high blood sugar, the _Islets of Langerhans_ release insulin into the bloodstream.

3. Glycogen is converted into glucose in a process known as _Glycogenolysis_

4. The loss of fluid from extracellular compartments is called _Osmotic diuresis_.

5. The condition known as polyuria suggests that there is an excessive production of _urine_.

6. A type of phenomenon in which the blood sugar levels rise between 5 A.M. and 8 A.M. is called _dawn phenomenon_

7. The classic three "Ps" of diabetes mellitus are _polyuria_, _polydipsia_, and _polyphagia_.

## MULTIPLE CHOICE

Circle the answer that best completes the following statements.

1. The nurse understands that the diabetic client must be cautious when exercising because:
   A. blood sugar levels may drop rapidly.
   B. hyperglycemia may develop.
   C. insulin dosages need to be increased.
   D. exercise produces fatigue and weakness.

2. The nurse is explaining the action of an oral antidiabetic agent. The best statement that reflects the nurse's understanding is as follows:
   A. The medication increases the production of natural insulin.
   B. Beta cells are stimulated to release more insulin in response to hyperglycemia.
   C. Oral agents provide long-acting release of previously injected pork insulin.
   D. Antidiabetic agents slow insulin production by the pancreas.

3. Jacob is being evaluated for possible diabetes mellitus. When collecting the initial data, the nurse should ask:
   A. "Do you eat a lot of sweets?"
   B. "How long have you been overweight?"
   C. "Do you have to urinate frequently?"
   D. "Have you had this type of blood work done before?"

4. The nurse is discussing hypoglycemic reactions with a family. Which of the following statements made by the spouse indicates further teaching is not needed?
   A. "I'll make sure that we have some hard candy at home."
   B. "The coffee will make him wake up real fast."
   C. "His son is going to pick up some hamburgers for later."
   D. "We have some wine in the refrigerator if he gets too sleepy."

5. A newly diagnosed patient with diabetes is concerned about his children. He asks if they should be tested for hyperglycemia. The nurse responds:
   A. "Probably; diabetes may be hereditary."
   B. "Yes, your children will have the same condition."
   C. "No, the disease is caused by a virus."
   D. "It's better to find out now than later."

6. A major characteristic found in insulin-dependent diabetes would include which of following?
   A. Generally resistant to the development of ketosis.
   B. Usually occurs before the age of 30.
   C. Pancreas produces small amount of insulin.
   D. Considered an autoimmune destruction of the alpha cells.

7. The nurse is teaching a class on the care of a diabetic patient. She states that early signs of diabetic ketoacidosis are:
   A. cool, clammy skin; nervousness.
   B. hunger, headache, tremors.
   C. dark, scanty urine and diarrhea.
   D. thirst, dry mucous membranes, poor skin turgor.

8. A vial of insulin is labeled U-100. The nurse recognizes this as:
   A. 100 mg/unit.
   B. 100 units/bottle.
   C. 100 units/dose.
   D. 100 units/mL.

9. If the nurse needs to decide how soon before a meal to give an insulin injection, which of the following must be considered?
   A. onset
   B. peak
   C. duration
   D. limit

10. A diabetic client is seated in the waiting area of your clinic. He begins to complain of nausea and hunger. You observe that he is sweating, experiencing a few chills, and has cool, pale skin. You recognize that this client may be experiencing:
    A. hypotension.
    B. hyperglycemia.
    C. hypoglycemia.
    D. hypocalcemia.

11. Which of the following is the correct procedure for mixing insulins?
    A. Inject air into NPH vial, inject air into regular vial, withdraw regular insulin first.
    B. Inject air into regular vial, inject air into NPH vial, withdraw NPH first.
    C. Withdraw regular insulin first, then withdraw NPH.
    D. Withdraw NPH first, then withdraw regular insulin.

12. A client is admitted to the hospital, diagnosed with type 2 diabetes mellitus, and scheduled for discharge the following day. The nurse realizes that the short hospital stay is not sufficient for adequate diabetic teaching; therefore, the client's education should:
    A. include specific, realistic goals.
    B. reflect a complete care plan that can be implanted by the home health nurse.
    C. be concise, comprehensive, and intense.
    D. involve the client's family only.

13. Mr. Jackson, diagnosed with type 2 DM, is prescribed an 1800-calorie diet with daily exercise. The client's assessment caring data include: T-98.6, P-90, R-20, BP-160/98, height – 5′5″, weight – 185 pounds. A dietary counseling referral was requested. The primary goal of nutritional therapy is:
    A. control of dietary intake to achieve ideal body weight.
    B. elimination of simple sugars.
    C. reduction in dietary calories to maintain normal blood pressure.
    D. daily equal distribution of carbohydrates.

14. A client has been seen by the diabetic nurse. You determine that additional teaching is necessary when the client says:
    A. "I may have an occasional beer if I include it in my meal plan."
    B. "I will need a bedtime snack."
    C. "I can eat as much as I want to as long as I cover it with additional insulin."
    D. "I should eat my meals, even if I am not hungry."

15. A 16-year-old male client has been using self-capillary blood glucose monitoring as part of his diabetic management. After evaluating his technique, the nurse identifies a need for additional teaching because the client:
    A. chose a puncture site in the center of the finger pad.
    B. washed his hands before the procedure.
    C. told the nurse that 110 mg/dL is a well-controlled value.
    D. disposes of the lancet in a sharps container.

## CRITICAL THINKING EXERCISE

Read the following situation. Unscramble the words and define each term. Answer the questions using the nursing process of assessment, diagnosis, planning, implementation, and evaluation.

An elderly client is admitted to your unit with a history of type 2 diabetes, *ripehalper asauclv seaseid* and *cerpglymyhia*. His vision is poor. During your assessment, you discover a 1-cm lesion on the bottom of the left heel. The client tells you that he had worn a new pair of shoes several days ago and the sore was not there at the time. The physician places the client on bed rest, *iiboticsant,* and a *diingls alecs* for insulin coverage.

1. List three predisposing factors that may have influenced the development of the decubitus ulcer.

2. Discuss the pathophysiology of the lesion.

3. Why did the physician order bed rest for this client?

4. The client's glucose is 200 mg/dL. Determine the amount of insulin you would give based on the ordered sliding scale: 300 or >, call the physician; 250–299, give 10 units regular insulin; 150–249, give 5 units regular insulin; <150, do not give insulin.

# Chapter 18

## The Gastrointestinal System and Assessment

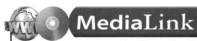

**www.prenhall.com/burke**

Use the address above to access the free, interactive Companion Website created for this textbook. Get hints, instant feedback, and textbook references to chapter-related NCLEX-style questions. Link to other interesting sites.

**Audio Glossary:**

Use the Companion Website, or the CD-ROM disk enclosed with your textbook, to hear the pronunciation of key terms in this chapter.

A healthy, well-balanced diet is necessary for proper body function. Food must be changed into a form that can supply energy for cell metabolism. The upper gastrointestinal system includes the mouth, esophagus, stomach, and small intestines. Each part has a role in digestion and the absorption of nutrients.

## GASTROINTESTINAL TERMINOLOGY

Match each term with its appropriate definition.

| | |
|---|---|
| 1. _____ GI tract | A. Metabolizes carbohydrates, proteins, and fats |
| 2. _____ Stomach | B. Carries food to the stomach |
| 3. _____ Parietal cell | C. Upper opening of the GI tract lined with mucous membranes |
| 4. _____ Chief cell | D. Secretes hormones that regulate digestion |
| 5. _____ Mucous cell | E. Continuous hollow tube |
| 6. _____ Enteroendocrine cell | F. Secretes hydrochloric acid and intrinsic factor |
| 7. _____ Liver | G. Contains amylase and lysozymes to break down food |
| 8. _____ Mouth | H. Protects the lining of the stomach from gastric juices |
| 9. _____ Saliva | I. Connected to the esophagus at the upper end and the small intestine at the lower end |
| 10. _____ Esophagus | J. Produces pepsin, which digests protein |

## FILL IN THE BLANK

Fill in the blanks with the appropriate word or phrase.

1. A client comes to the clinic complaining of severe abdominal pain that started today. As you ask about his current medication history the client states, "Well, I've had a headache for two days that I can't seem to get rid of, and I've tried everything." You suspect the client has been using _____.

2. You are out to lunch with a friend when she frowns and states, "I need to go to the doctor! This heartburn is starting to bother me!" You suspect that her _____, normally closed except during swallowing, is malfunctioning.

3. The nervous system (parasympathetic) stimulates gastric secretion via the _____.

4. A client, 72 years of age, has had several nutritional education referrals for his anorexia. He is 5′11″ and weighs 145 pounds. He says, "I'm just not hungry." You know that any change in gastrointestinal function with aging has a significant effect on _____, general health, and well-being.

5. A flexible tube used to visualize the GI tract is called a _____.

## MULTIPLE CHOICE

Circle the answer that best completes the following statements.

1. A patient suffering from multiple dental caries states, "I've been dieting a lot lately." What type of diet is this patient on?
   A. high carbohydrates
   B. low fat
   C. high protein
   D. fasting

2. Dianne, a patient in the hospital, has not eaten well in several days. She and her boyfriend broke up before she entered the hospital. The nurse realizes that emotions such as stress or anxiety affect the GI tract by:
   A. increasing gastric secretions.
   B. neutralizing stomach acid.
   C. inhibiting gastric motility.
   D. excreting bile.

3. The nurse is caring for a patient with liver cancer. Her main concern at this time would be:
   A. prevention of constipation.
   B. prevention of infection.
   C. prevention of gastric reflux.
   D. prevention of discomfort.

4. A gastric analysis includes which of the following?
   A. allowing the patient to smoke
   B. inserting an NG tube
   C. observing for falls
   D. comparing preanalysis weight

5. Bill is 6′0″ and weighs 230 pounds. According to the weight chart he should weigh about 185 pounds. Bill is considered to be:
   A. within the normal range.
   B. overweight.
   C. obese.
   D. morbidly obese.

6. Corey was admitted with diarrhea and dehydration. He has at least four foul-smelling, mucous-filled loose stools every 3 hours. You know the doctor will order a:
   A. serum albumin level.
   B. gastric lavage.
   C. endoscopy.
   D. specimen for ova and parasites.

7. You are explaining smoking cessation to a patient diagnosed with pancreatic disease. Your best explanation might be:
   A. "The tar in the cigarette coats the lining of the stomach."
   B. "Smoking increases the production of gastric acid secretion."
   C. "Cigarettes inhibit bicarbonate secretion."
   D. "The nicotine increases blood flow to the gastric mucosa."

8. Mr. Lee, an 89-year-old patient who rarely eats his meals, is losing weight. The nurse knows to assess:
   A. mucous membranes and gums.
   B. food tolerance.
   C. A and B.
   D. B only.

9. Ms. Ray has soft, spoon-shaped nails. The nurse is aware that this is due to:
   A. protein deficiency.
   B. high-fat diet.
   C. smoking.
   D. iron deficiency.

10. Mrs. Matherly is returning to your unit following a lower GI series. Which of the following nursing interventions is the most important?
    A. Encourage fluids.
    B. Monitor for pain.
    C. Provide detailed postop instructions.
    D. Encourage splinting.

## CRITICAL THINKING EXERCISE

Read the following situation. Unscramble the words and define each term. Answer the questions using the nursing process of assessment, diagnosis, planning, implementation, and evaluation.

A 25-year-old female is being prepared for a(n) *dlaamiobn dutralounds* in the morning. She has been diagnosed with acute *iittsrsag* caused by the *lltonagsste*. The nurse reviews her chart and notes that she has been *tvoinmg* after meals.

1. Name the primary nursing diagnosis that would be appropriate at this time.

2. Discuss the diet appropriate for this patient.

3. Name three teaching interventions that you would initiate before the procedure.

# Chapter 19

# Caring for Clients with Nutritional and Upper Gastrointestinal Disorders

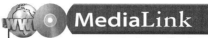

## MediaLink

**www.prenhall.com/burke**

Use the address above to access the free, interactive Companion Website created for this textbook. Get hints, instant feedback, and textbook references to chapter-related NCLEX-style questions. Link to other interesting sites.

**Audio Glossary:**

Use the Companion Website, or the CD-ROM disk enclosed with your textbook, to hear the pronunciation of key terms in this chapter.

A healthy, well-balanced diet is necessary for proper body function. When caring for patients with nutritional or gastrointestinal disorders, it is important to give them the information they need to help their bodies maintain a sense of balance or to seek professional help when necessary.

## GASTROINTESTINAL TERMINOLOGY

Match each term with its appropriate definition.

1. _____ Chyme
2. _____ Hematemesis
3. _____ Nutrition
4. _____ Nutrient
5. _____ Malnutrition
6. _____ Melena
7. _____ Metabolism
8. _____ Peristalsis
9. _____ Dysphagia
10. _____ Small intestine

A. Physical and chemical processes of cell activity
B. Waves of contractions found in GI tract
C. Bloody emesis
D. Pain or difficulty swallowing
E. Substances needed for growth, maintenance, and repair
F. Properties of food that build healthy bodies
G. Poor nourishment from improper diet or metabolic defect
H. Blood in the stool
I. Chemically breaks down and absorbs food
J. Partially digested food with gastric juices

## FILL IN THE BLANK

Fill in the blanks with the appropriate word or phrase.

1. A client comes to the clinic for a routine exam. During your interview, he asks you about over-the-counter "stomach remedies." He admits that the Pepsid and antacids he bought have not helped his stomach pains. He has lost 10 pounds within the last 3 months. His medical records indicate that he has been treated for *H. pylori* on three occasions. You suspect that this client may be diagnosed with a form of _____.

2. A neighbor drops by your house and asks you what to do about the white patches that have developed in her mouth. She states that she cannot eat because of the pain. She also tells you that she is being treated for a bacterial infection but the antibiotics don't seem to be helping. You suspect that her primary physician will make the diagnosis of _____.

3. Mr. Jones, 42-year-old executive, presents in the ED with severe burning sensations in his chest. Vital signs are T-99.1, P-90, R-22, BP-150/88. As the physician enters the room, Mr. Jones cries out in pain, holding his abdomen and sweating profusely. Bowel sounds are absent. The physician immediately suspects _____.

4. A client, 24 years of age, has had several nutritional education referrals for her obesity. She is 5′5″ and weighs 300 pounds. She says that she is always hungry and is not able to stay on any prescribed diet. This client's primary nursing diagnosis should be _____.

5. Mr. Kinard comes to the clinic complaining of stomach problems. He states that he eats Tums antacids as if they were candy. The doctor suspects that Mr. Kinard has an ulcer and schedules him for a _____.

6. A client schedules a visit with his physician to discuss his chest and stomach discomfort. He indicates that the pain is in the substernal area and that he is unable to lie down after eating. He also complains of a burning fluid in his throat at bedtime. Based on this information, the nurse can anticipate that this client will be treated for _____.

7. To maintain the nitrogen balance in the body and to build muscle, it is necessary to eat a diet high in _____.

## MULTIPLE CHOICE

Circle the answer that best completes the following statements.

1. A patient suffering from bulimia is at risk for:
   A. weight gain.
   B. diarrhea.
   C. esophageal damage.
   D. hyperglycemia.

2. Johnny is going to be receiving enteral tube feedings for a period of time. You know that enteral feedings may be administered through:
   A. nasogastric and gastric tubes.
   B. gastric and cecum tubes.
   C. gastric tubes only.
   D. nasogastric, gastrostomy, and jejunostomy tubes.

3. The nurse is caring for a stroke patient receiving 120 mL Ensure/hour. Her main concern at this time would be:
   A. prevention of diarrhea.
   B. prevention of aspiration.
   C. prevention of nasal irritation.
   D. prevention of constipation.

4. A client receiving TPN would be expected to have daily blood specimens drawn for:
   A. calcium.
   B. glucose.
   C. sodium.
   D. potassium.

5. Mary is 5′6″ and weighs 160 pounds. According to the weight chart she should weigh about 145 pounds. Mary is considered to be:
   A. within the normal range.
   B. overweight.
   C. obese.
   D. morbidly obese.

6. Maxine was admitted with acute gastritis. During her morning bath, she suddenly begins to throw up blood. Your first action should be to:
   A. administer prescribed antiemetic.
   B. raise the head of the bed.
   C. increase the IV fluid rate.
   D. call the physician.

7. You are explaining to a patient who has been diagnosed with peptic ulcer disease the effects of cigarette smoking on the stomach. Your best explanation might be:
   A. "The tar in the cigarette coats the lining of the stomach."
   B. "Smoking increases the production of gastric acid secretion."
   C. "Cigarettes inhibit bicarbonate secretion."
   D. "The nicotine increases blood flow to the gastric mucosa."

8. Mr. Jessup tells you that he becomes nauseated about 10 minutes after he has eaten. In addition, he states that his stomach cramps and makes loud noises. To alleviate some of these symptoms, the nurse would suggest:
   A. Eat two large meals a day.
   B. Drink lots of water with the food.
   C. Rest in a recumbent position after eating.
   D. Increase the amount of simple sugars in the diet.

9. The nurse is aware that there is an increased risk for stomach cancer in clients who:
    A. eat diets high in fiber.
    B. have been diagnosed with *H. pylori*.
    C. are under a lot of stress.
    D. smoke two packs of cigarettes per day.

10. Mrs. Elliot is returning to your unit following an endoscopy. Which of the following nursing interventions is the most important?
    A. Withhold fluids until the gag reflex returns.
    B. Monitor for pain.
    C. Provide detailed discharge instructions.
    D. Discourage coughing.

11. You are performing a gastric lavage and have suctioned 135 mL of fluids from the stomach. Your initial irrigation was 100 mL of water. On the I&O record you will document:
    A. 135 mL gastric contents.
    B. 235 mL gastric contents and lavage.
    C. 35 mL gastric contents.
    D. 100 mL gastric contents.

12. Mrs. Tubbman has a new gastrostomy tube that is going to be used for the first time. You are unable to aspirate any stomach contents. Bowel sounds are absent. Your next action is to:
    A. use the tube because the x-ray verified placement.
    B. hold the tube feeding until the doctor makes rounds.
    C. call the doctor and inform him of your findings.
    D. ask the charge nurse to begin the feedings.

13. You are teaching a client about the use of metoclopramide. Which of the following is not true concerning this medication?
    A. May cause drowsiness.
    B. Used to prevent dizzy spells.
    C. Adverse reactions with alcohol have been documented.
    D. May have a side effect of muscle tremors.

14. The school nurse is seeing an 18-year-old girl for complaints of fatigue. The client states that her vitamins "just don't seem to work." She appears unusually thin. The nurse believes that the client needs further teaching because:
    A. teenagers are not nutritionally educated.
    B. teen girls are at risk for poor nutrition due to societal expectations.
    C. she is on the basketball team and weight loss is expected.
    D. she is not taking the proper amount of vitamins.

15. Measures that are used to evaluate obesity include:
    A. BMI.
    B. fat-fold.
    C. bioelectrical impedance.
    D. all of the above.

## CRITICAL THINKING EXERCISE

Read the following situation. Unscramble the words and define each term. Answer the questions using the nursing process of assessment, diagnosis, planning, implementation, and evaluation.

A 47-year-old male is being prepared for a *trospycosag* in the morning. He has been diagnosed with acute *iittsrsag* caused by the *licoretbacHe loriyp* organism. The nurse reviews his chart and notes that he has been using *AIDSSN* for back pain.

1. Name the primary nursing diagnosis that would be appropriate at this time.
2. Discuss the teaching required for this procedure.
3. Name three interventions that you would initiate after the procedure.
4. What information should be documented regarding his scheduled test?

# Chapter 20

## Caring for Clients with Bowel Disorders

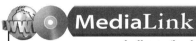

**MediaLink**

**www.prenhall.com/burke**

Use the address above to access the free, interactive Companion Website created for this textbook. Get hints, instant feedback, and textbook references to chapter-related NCLEX-style questions. Link to other interesting sites.

**Audio Glossary:**

Use the Companion Website, or the CD-ROM disk enclosed with your textbook, to hear the pronunciation of key terms in this chapter.

The digestion and synthesis of food is the purpose of the small intestine. Excess water and wastes are eliminated from the gastrointestinal tract via the large intestine. Any disruption of these processes results in potential debilitating and life-threatening complications for the client.

## ANATOMY AND PHYSIOLOGY

Match each term with its appropriate definition.

1. _____ Duodenum
2. _____ Chyme
3. _____ Ileocecal valve
4. _____ Sigmoid colon
5. _____ Feces
6. _____ Defecation reflex
7. _____ Valsalva's
8. _____ Goblet cells
9. _____ Appendix
10. _____ Anus

A. Located in the intestinal tract and produces mucus
B. Outlet of the rectum
C. First part of the large intestine
D. Body waste
E. Mixture of partly digested food and digestive secretions
F. Bearing-down movement
G. Worm-shaped pouch extending from the cecum
H. Connects the small and large intestines
I. Stimulation of stretch receptors to allow evacuation
J. S-shaped portion at the end of the descending colon

## FILL IN THE BLANK

Fill in the blanks with the appropriate word or phrase.

1. A client is admitted to the hospital for hypokalemia and dehydration. The most common cause of this condition is _____.

2. The physician's orders include an upper GI and barium enema for a client experiencing alterations in diarrhea and constipation, lower abdominal pain, and excessive mucous production. The most probable diagnosis for this client is _____.

3. Mr. Chen, 42 years old, tells the nurse that he is not able to eat many of the commercial cereals. He states that his father had the same condition. The nurse anticipates that the physician will diagnose Mr. Chen with _____.

4. A 14-year-old female is admitted to the medical floor with severe right lower abdominal pain. Her temperature is 101°F. Rebound tenderness is noted during palpation. This client probably has _____.

5. The nurse is assessing a male patient who complains that he "got sick after he ate at a local restaurant." Objective data include a loss of 350 mL of emesis and 400 mL of watery stool. This client is exhibiting signs of _____.

6. A 27-year-old client has been experiencing attacks of diarrhea with some rectal bleeding over the last year. She has become weak and anorexic. The diagnosis that the physician will write in his notes will probably be _____.

7. A 72-year-old male has presented to the clinic with complaints of unusual stools with bleeding on occasion. His hemoglobin is low. The doctor suspects that this client may have colon _____.

## MULTIPLE CHOICE

Circle the answer that best completes the following statements.

1. The nurse is changing an ostomy pouch. Which of the following should be completed first?
   A. Note the color of the stoma and surrounding skin.
   B. Use a measuring guide to check stoma size.
   C. Remove the soiled pouch.
   D. Cleanse the skin with soap and water.

2. You are assisting an elderly client in filling out the diet menu. The client has chronic diarrhea. Which of the following items should not be ordered for this client?
   A. apple juice
   B. roast beef
   C. green beans
   D. spaghetti

3. The nurse would question the medication order for a patient taking a monoamine oxidase inhibitor if which of the following were added to the medication record?
   A. Pepto-Bismol
   B. Lomotil
   C. Sandostatin
   D. Dipentum

4. A young client asks the nurse what causes constipation. The best response is:
   A. lack of exercise.
   B. chronic laxative use.
   C. voluntary suppression of the urge.
   D. all of the above.

5. A patient is preparing for a colonoscopy. The physician orders magnesium citrate. Which of the following statements, if made by the patient, indicates an understanding of your teaching instructions?
   A. "I'll take the medication at bedtime so it has time to work."
   B. "If I keep the drink at room temperature it will taste better."
   C. "This medication will give me some cramps."
   D. "It's okay to eat breakfast at 6 A.M., since my exam isn't until 8 A.M."

6. An elderly client has been taking mineral oil as a laxative routinely for several months. The nurse can expect that this client will have a deficiency of:
   A. vitamin A.
   B. vitamin C.
   C. vitamin B.
   D. vitamin F.

7. When preparing a client for a sigmoidoscopy, the teaching plan should include which of the following instructions?
   A. Sterile water may be injected into the bowel for better visualization.
   B. The client will be placed in the prone position.
   C. No food or water can be consumed 8 hours before the test.
   D. The procedure will take about 15 minutes.

8. The primary purpose for assessing the patency of a nasogastric tube is to:
   A. prevent aspiration pneumonia.
   B. remove gastrointestinal secretions.
   C. assess for the return of peristalsis.
   D. replace electrolytes.

9. Which of the following clients is at high risk for developing colon cancer?
   A. 58-year-old male diagnosed with prostate cancer
   B. 24-year-old female with a family history of ovarian cancer
   C. 37-year-old male with inflammatory bowel disease
   D. 16-year-old female with morbid obesity

10. A client tells you that his colostomy bag odor is embarrassing and asks you what he can do to minimize this problem. Your best response should be:
    A. "Be sure to eat lots of cabbage and eggs."
    B. "There's not much that we can do about the smell."
    C. "There are odor tablets that you can put in the bag."
    D. "I don't think the smell is so bad. Don't worry about it."

11. Which observation of a client who has a nursing diagnosis of Risk for Impaired Skin Integrity would indicate that the outcome is successful?
    A. Client has developed a small, 2-cm reddened area on his sacrum.
    B. Client has a small rash on the perineal area.
    C. Client's skin is intact.
    D. Client requires aloe vera cream for lesion on buttocks.

12. When a client has a nursing diagnosis of Risk for Deficient Fluid Volume, which of the following nursing interventions should be included on the care plan?
    A. Maintain accurate intake and output records.
    B. Record the client's weight weekly.
    C. Assess for signs of dehydration, such as moist skin.
    D. Document the vital signs every shift.

13. Which of the following nursing diagnoses would be the most appropriate for a client with colon cancer?
    A. Acute Pain
    B. Anticipatory Grieving
    C. Risk for Sexual Dysfunction
    D. Risk for Impaired Skin Integrity

14. A client is being discharged from the hospital with a new ostomy appliance. Prior to discharge, it is important to request a referral to the:
    A. dietitian.
    B. home health nurse.
    C. ostomy and wound care nurse.
    D. physical therapist.

15. A 24-year-old client is admitted to the surgical floor with excruciating pain in the right groin. He is nauseated and has vomited 300 mL of yellow bile. Visible inspection reveals a mass in the groin. The medical diagnosis for this client might be:
    A. ventral hernia.
    B. strangulated hernia.
    C. umbilical hernia.
    D. incisional hernia.

## CRITICAL THINKING EXERCISE

Read the following situation. Unscramble the words and define each term. Answer the questions using the nursing process of assessment, diagnosis, planning, implementation, and evaluation.

A 24-year-old client is admitted to the same-day surgery unit for a *droitmorehechomy*. He had previously undergone *tagdiil neocdutri* and *therapyerocls,* both of which were unsuccessful. After the procedure, the physician orders a *zits* bath.

1. Discuss pain control for this client after his surgery.
2. Name three things that should be taught to prevent the recurrence of his hemorrhoids.
3. What information should be provided to this client regarding the recovery period?
4. Document the assessment after the patient returns from surgery.

# Chapter 21

## Caring for Clients with Gallbladder, Liver, and Pancreatic Disorders

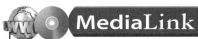

### MediaLink

**www.prenhall.com/burke**

Use the address above to access the free, interactive Companion Website created for this textbook. Get hints, instant feedback, and textbook references to chapter-related NCLEX-style questions. Link to other interesting sites.

**Audio Glossary:**

Use the Companion Website, or the CD-ROM disk enclosed with your textbook, to hear the pronunciation of key terms in this chapter.

Accessory disorders of the digestive system are intricately woven together. Even though these organs are separate, they affect the function of the other members. Clients with digestive disorders are unable to eat and thus suffer the problems of nutritional deficits.

## ANATOMY AND PHYSIOLOGY

Match each term with its appropriate definition.

| | | |
|---|---|---|
| 1. _____ Visceral | A. | Circular muscle found in bile duct |
| 2. _____ Hepatocytes | B. | Storage place for bile |
| 3. _____ Kupffer | C. | Liver cell |
| 4. _____ Sphincter of Oddi | D. | A salt that neutralizes acid |
| 5. _____ Lipase | E. | Phagocytic cell in the liver |
| 6. _____ Exocrine | F. | Yellow-orange fluid produced in liver |
| 7. _____ Bile | G. | Pertaining to any large organ in abdomen |
| 8. _____ Gallbladder | H. | Small vascular units in the liver |
| 9. _____ Lobules | I. | Fat-splitting enzyme |
| 10. _____ Bicarbonate | J. | Gland that secretes via a duct |

## FILL IN THE BLANK

Fill in the blanks with the appropriate word or phrase.

1. Mrs. Patience, age 48, is seen in your clinic with pain in the right upper quadrant with radiating pain to the right scapula. She has been nauseated and unable to eat for several days. The physician orders a HIDA scan. Based on this information, you suspect the client will be treated for

   _____.

2.  An outbreak of hepatitis has occurred in a small Third World country. The living conditions are unsanitary and the food is poorly prepared. The most likely type of hepatitis might be _____.

3.  A 58-year-old homeless man is brought to the emergency department. He has a history of alcohol abuse and hepatitis. This form of hepatitis is classified as _____.

4.  Mrs. Baskins is admitted to your unit with varicosities of the esophagus. The initial assessment reveals ascites, splenomegaly, and portal hypertension. You suspect that this client will be diagnosed with _____.

5.  The nurse is reviewing the chart of a patient admitted from the emergency department. The physical exam indicates that the patient has decreased mental abilities and motor function and has been in liver failure for several weeks. When she observes him for the first time, she notes that his hands are flapping. The diagnosis for this patient is most likely _____.

6.  A client with chronic hepatitis B has been taken to surgery for a liver biopsy. The physical assessment reveals hepatomegaly with a large mass in the outer edge and severe jaundice. The nurse suspects that the physician believes that this client may have liver _____.

7.  The physician has requested the nurse to prepare a consent form for a client with pancreatic cancer. She anticipates that this type of surgical procedure will be a _____.

## MULTIPLE CHOICE

Circle the answer that best completes the following statements.

1.  You are discussing the various forms of hepatitis with the nursing instructor. She asks you which viral hepatitis is transmitted only by blood. Your response should be:
    A.  G.
    B.  E.
    C.  D.
    D.  C.

2.  Which prescription would the nurse anticipate for a client who has been diagnosed with cirrhosis of the liver?
    A.  lactulose
    B.  acetaminophen
    C.  ibuprophen
    D.  Demerol

3.  As a result of a client's positive HIDA scan, the nurse expects his immediate treatment to include:
    A.  high-protein diet.
    B.  low-protein diet.
    C.  high-fat diet.
    D.  low-fat diet.

4. A client has been diagnosed with acute pancreatitis. Which of the following complications should be anticipated by the nurse?
   A. hypertension
   B. flank bruising
   C. hypoglycemia
   D. fever

5. Mr. Blue, 48 years old, is diagnosed with cirrhosis of the liver. Which intervention should the nurse plan to include in the client's skin care?
   A. Rub the skin briskly to aid in the drying process.
   B. Turn the client every 20 minutes.
   C. Use hot water when bathing.
   D. Avoid soap for bathing.

6. You are preparing a client for a paracentesis. Which of the following best explains the procedure?
   A. Fluid is removed from the retroperitoneal cavity.
   B. A long needle is inserted into the retroperitoneal cavity.
   C. A needle is inserted into the peritoneal cavity and fluid is withdrawn.
   D. Fluid is removed from the thoracic cavity by a long needle.

7. The nurse is reviewing the lab results for a client with acute pancreatitis. Which of the following would verify that this diagnosis is correct?
   A. serum amylase 184 U/L
   B. serum lipase 10 U/L
   C. serum calcium 12 mg/dL
   D. WBC 5500

8. A client is receiving spironolactone for treatment of cirrhosis. Which of the following statements, if made by the client, would indicate that he understands the medication teaching?
   A. "I'm going to report any diarrhea to my doctor."
   B. "I should take this medication in the morning."
   C. "If I have any ringing in the ears, I'll call you."
   D. "I'll weigh myself every other day."

9. A client returns from surgery with a T-tube. Which of the following interventions would not be appropriate for this client?
   A. Place in Fowler's position.
   B. Keep the T-tube clamped.
   C. Monitor color and consistency of drainage.
   D. Assess skin for bile leakage.

10. When assessing a client in the preicteric phase of acute viral hepatitis, the nurse would expect to identify which of these symptoms?
    A. pruritus
    B. clay-colored stools
    C. flulike symptoms
    D. increased energy

11. A patient with acute hepatitis is experiencing anorexia and nausea. These signs would substantiate a nursing diagnosis of:
    A. Self-Care Deficit.
    B. Activity Intolerance.
    C. Risk for Infection.
    D. Altered Nutrition: Less than Body Requirements.

12. Which of these events, if present in a patient's history, is most likely related to the development of hepatitis?
    A. injection drug user
    B. recent travel to Florida
    C. viral infection of the upper airway
    D. history of flu vaccine

13. You are assisting in a liver biopsy. If all of the following are postprocedure nursing interventions, which should be your highest priority?
    A. Position the client on his right side.
    B. Keep NPO for 2 hours.
    C. Frequently assess site.
    D. Apply direct pressure after the needle is removed.

14. The nurse is teaching a client about the importance of bleeding precautions. Which of the following should not be included in the care plan?
    A. Avoid blowing nose.
    B. Use a medium-hard toothbrush.
    C. Assess for purpura.
    D. Avoid injections.

15. Lactulose is frequently used in the treatment of hepatic encephalopathy. The purpose of this medication is to:
    A. inhibit ammonia absorption in the bowel.
    B. destroy intestinal bacteria.
    C. reduce ascites.
    D. reduce peristalsis.

## CRITICAL THINKING EXERCISE

Read the following situation. Unscramble the words and define each term. Answer the questions using the nursing process of assessment, diagnosis, planning, implementation, and evaluation.

Mr. Seawell, 47 years old, has been admitted to the hospital for *holicoalc patehitis*. He has *dicenaunj* and complains of nausea. The physician has ordered a *rumes lasymae* and a *centrasisaep* procedure kit to the bedside.

1. What condition is commonly seen as a result of alcoholic hepatitis?
2. Name three nursing actions that should be completed before the paracentesis.
3. Discuss the diet that should be provided for this client.
4. Document the paracentesis in the nursing notes.

# Chapter 22

# The Respiratory System and Assessment

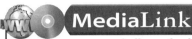

**www.prenhall.com/burke**

Use the address above to access the free, interactive Companion Website created for this textbook. Get hints, instant feedback, and textbook references to chapter-related NCLEX-style questions. Link to other interesting sites.

**Audio Glossary:**

Use the Companion Website, or the CD-ROM disk enclosed with your textbook, to hear the pronunciation of key terms in this chapter.

The primary function of the respiratory system is to provide the cells of the body with oxygen and to eliminate carbon dioxide (a waste product of cellular metabolism). Nursing assessment of respiratory function is vital in clients with disorders and diseases affecting the respiratory system, as well as in clients at risk for respiratory complications of other disorders. It is a particularly important component when assessing older adults.

## ANATOMY AND PHYSIOLOGY

Match each term with its appropriate definition.

1. __B__ Vocal cords
2. __I__ Eustachian tubes
3. __H__ Nares
4. __D__ Nasopharynx
5. __J__ Epiglottis
6. __A__ Larynx
7. __E__ Turbinates
8. __F__ Sinuses
9. __C__ Nasal hairs
10. __G__ Soft palate

A. Located between laryngopharynx and trachea

B. Mucous membranes that produce speech

C. Filter air as it enters the nose

D. Contains the tonsils and adenoids

E. Traps large particles within nasal cavity

F. Openings in facial bones that lighten the skull

G. Prevents food from entering nasopharynx

H. External opening of nasal cavity

I. Connects middle ear and nasopharynx

J. Closes during swallowing to prevent aspiration

## FILL IN THE BLANK

Fill in the blanks with the appropriate word or phrase.

1. Nancy was choking in the restaurant when someone administered the Heimlich maneuver. Instead of coughing up whatever she was choking on, Nancy became unconscious. Someone yelled, "Stick your finger down her throat to make her throw up!" You know this won't work because _Cough Reflex doesn't work when unconscious_

2. _Ventilation_ air movement into and out of the lungs, has two phases: *inspiration,* as air flows into the lungs, and *expiration,* when gases flow out of the lungs.

3. Breathing is controlled by respiratory centers in the brain and by _Chemoreceptors_ in the brain, aortic arch, and carotid arteries.

4. _Compliance_ depends on both lung tissue and the rib cage.

5. The loss of elasticity in aging increases the residual volume of the lungs and reduces vital capacity. As a result of these changes, the client is at greater risk for developing respiratory infections and being unable to effectively clear _secretions_ from the alveoli and airways.

6. Abnormal breath sounds are also known as _adventitious_ breath sounds.

7. A noninvasive test, often used to evaluate and monitor oxygen saturation ($SaO_2$) of blood in clients with respiratory disorders is called _pulse ox_.

## MULTIPLE CHOICE

Circle the answer that best completes the following statements.

1. The primary laboratory tests used to evaluate the respiratory system and diagnose disorders affecting it are:
   A. tissue biopsy, pulse oximetry, arterial blood gases.
   B. arterial blood gases, tissue biopsy, and nasal, throat, and sputum cultures.
   C. nasal, throat, and sputum cultures, ear swab, tissue biopsy.
   D. tissue biopsy, arterial blood gases, blood glucose.

2. Tissue for biopsy, or microscopic examination, may be obtained by needle aspiration of a:
   A. lymph node.
   B. brain cell.
   C. spinal membrane.
   D. bronchus.

3. Lung volume and capacity are measured with:
   A. LCDs.
   B. PETs.
   C. LATs.
   D. PFTs.

4. You are teaching a client going for a pulmonary function test to stop using bronchodilators, drinking caffeinated beverages, or smoking 4–6 hours before the test because:
   A. they could die.
   B. testing policy dictates.
   C. bronchodilators, smoking, and caffeine interfere with test results.
   D. the results will always be positive.

5. Marta, age 25, has asthma. She uses a peak expiratory flow rate (PEFR) meter on a day-to-day basis to:
   A. monitor air humidity.
   B. assess her breathing pattern.
   C. monitor airway constriction.
   D. balance the amount of rest periods and activities.

6. Jason, age 38, was diagnosed with laryngeal tumors via:
   A. laryngoscopy.
   B. bronchoscopy.
   C. EGD.
   D. EEG.

7. A patent airway and unobstructed airflow are vital to sustain life and:
   A. well-being.
   B. lung capacity.
   C. function.
   D. love.

8. Before doing a CT of the head and neck, an important nursing implication is to inquire about:
   A. consent.
   B. next of kin.
   C. bleeding.
   D. allergies.

9. Following arterial puncture, the nurse often is responsible for applying pressure to the site for a period of:
   A. 5 to 10 minutes.
   B. 30 minutes.
   C. 2 to 5 minutes.
   D. 1 hour.

10. A detergent-like substance that helps keep alveoli open is called:
    A. mainstem.
    B. hilus.
    C. surfactant.
    D. bronchus.

## CRITICAL THINKING EXERCISE

Read the following situation. Unscramble the words and define each term. Answer the questions using the nursing process of assessment, diagnosis, planning, implementation, and evaluation.

A patent airway and unobstructed airflow are vital to sustain *file* and function. The upper *ysirrpretao* system provides a passageway for air to the *slnug,* cleaning, humidifying, and warming the air that passes through it. Mucus and lymphoid tissue in the upper airway trap dust and bacteria, reducing the risk of lower airway contamination. The lungs and *irbonhc* of the lower respiratory system work together with the *nypaumrol* vessels in the process of respiration, which includes ventilation (breathing) and gas exchange in the alveoli.

1. Discuss the process of respiration.
2. What are the mechanics of respiration?
3. Discuss factors affecting respiration.

# Chapter 23

# Caring for Clients with Upper Respiratory Disorders

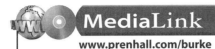

**www.prenhall.com/burke**

Use the address above to access the free, interactive Companion Website created for this textbook. Get hints, instant feedback, and textbook references to chapter-related NCLEX-style questions. Link to other interesting sites.

**Audio Glossary:**

Use the Companion Website, or the CD-ROM disk enclosed with your textbook, to hear the pronunciation of key terms in this chapter.

The respiratory system is designed for the process of inhalation of air into the lungs and the exhalation of carbon dioxide and other elements to the outside environment. The components of the upper respiratory tract warm the air, provide moisture, and serve as a protective mechanism against invading organisms.

## ANATOMY AND PHYSIOLOGY

Match each term with its appropriate definition.

1. D  Rhinitis
2. B  Influenza
3. E  Sinusitis
4. I  Pharyngitis
5. F  Tonsillitis

6. A  Otalgia
7. G  Stridor

8. C  Aphonia

9. H  Echinacea
10. J  Dyspnea

A.  Pain in the ear
B.  A highly contagious viral respiratory disease
C.  Complete loss of the voice
D.  Inflammation of the nasal cavities
E.  Inflammation of the mucous membranes of the sinuses
F.  Acute inflammation of the tonsils
G.  A high-pitched, harsh sound heard during inspiration
H.  Herbal remedy that may reduce the duration and symptoms of a common cold or influenza
I.  Acute inflammation of the throat
J.  Difficult or labored breathing

## FILL IN THE BLANK

Fill in the blanks with the appropriate word or phrase.

1. The patient, a 21-year-old music major, has presented in your clinic with complaints of a sore, swollen throat. He speaks in a very low voice and states that he cannot talk very loud. During your assessment you ask him when the problem first appeared. He tells you that he had just returned from a three-day choral concert in which he was the lead singer. You suspect that this patient is experiencing _laryngitis_.

2. During the initial assessment, the nurse obtains the following objective data: T-101.8, BP-132/68, R-24, P-98. The patient complains of dysphagia and throat pain. The physician orders a throat culture for strep. Based on these findings you believe that the patient may have _pharyngitis_.

3. You are examining the throat of a 14-year-old male patient and note that the tonsils are swollen, red, and filled with purulent exudate. In addition, the patient complains of otalgia and a "tired" feeling. These findings may indicate the presence of _tonsilitis_. The physician also determines that the patient has pus behind the tonsils and detects that the uvula has deviated to the left side. This condition is referred to as _acute epiglotitis_

4. You are working in a family practice clinic. A 10-year-old patient is brought into the clinic with breathing difficulties, including restlessness, stridor, and nasal flaring. The patient's mother reports that the child has had a severe sore throat for several days, has not attended classes at school, and has refused to eat due to swallowing problems. You recognize that this is a medical emergency which was brought about by the probable diagnosis of

   _____.

5. You are caring for an 80-year-old female with the following signs and symptoms: T-101.2, chills, coryza, fatigue, substernal burning. Your nursing instructor asks you which of the following may be affecting your patient: acute viral rhinitis, allergic rhinitis, influenza. You reply that the patient may be experiencing _____.

6. A patient complains of itchy, watery eyes, headache, runny nose, and frequent episodes of sneezing. During the assessment, you discover that the patient has recently been employed as a dog groomer at the local pet shop. She states that she rarely "gets a cold." You suspect that the patient may be experiencing _____.

7. A patient presents to the emergency department with dizziness, severe headaches in the forehead, purulent nasal discharge, and a foul odor in the mouth. This patient may be diagnosed by the physician with

   _____.

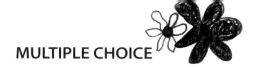
Circle the answer that best completes the following statements.

1.  Before administering the polyvalent influenza virus vaccine to a patient, the nurse should:
    A.  ask the patient about previous flu episodes.
    B.  obtain vital signs.
    C.  note patient allergies to eggs.
    D.  request the patient to sign an informed consent.

2.  The patient who is receiving antibiotics for a bacterial infection is no longer contagious after:
    A.  12 hours.
    B.  24 hours.
    C.  48 hours.
    D.  72 hours.

3.  Which of the following medications, if used longer than 3 to 5 days, may result in rebound congestion?
    A.  fexofenadine
    B.  Neo-Synephrine
    C.  clesmastine
    D.  Allegra

4.  You are assigned to assist in writing the discharge plans for a patient who has had endoscopic sinus surgery. Patient teaching should include:
    A.  sneeze into a tissue to prevent spreading of microorganisms.
    B.  no lifting restrictions after 3 days.
    C.  avoid smoking.
    D.  notify the physician for a temperature greater than 100°F.

5.  Nursing interventions for the diagnosis of Ineffective Airway Clearance should include:
    A.  balance the amount of rest periods and activities.
    B.  assess the patient's sleep patterns.
    C.  monitor the cough reflex.
    D.  instruct the patient in the use of throat lozenges.

6.  Posterior nosebleeds are usually associated with secondary systemic disorders. The individual most affected by this form of epistaxis is the:
    A.  30-year-old football player.
    B.  62-year-old housewife.
    C.  14-year-old ballet dancer.
    D.  76-year-old retired engineer.

7.  Appropriate first aid for the patient with an anterior nosebleed includes:
    A.  pinching the nose away from the septum.
    B.  applying ice packs to the nose.
    C.  sitting position, leaning slightly backward.
    D.  tilting the head upward.

8. The most common broken bone of the face is the:
   A. mandible.
   B. maxilla.
   C. nose.
   D. temporal bone.

9. Your patient has undergone rhinoplasty and will be discharged from the hospital in 2 days. He is anxious about the swelling and bruising on his face and asks how long the bruises will be noticeable. You reply that this condition should subside in:
   A. 3–5 days.
   B. 6–10 days.
   C. 10–14 days.
   D. several months.

10. The most common cause of airway obstruction in the adult is:
    A. swollen tongue.
    B. drowning.
    C. anaphylactic shock.
    D. food lodged in the throat.

11. The term used to describe a high-pitched, wheezing sound created by an airway obstruction is called:
    A. crowing.
    B. stridor.
    C. sonorous.
    D. crepitus.

12. Upper airway tumors are most commonly found in the:
    A. trachea.
    B. larynx.
    C. nasopharynx.
    D. oropharynx.

13. Laryngeal cancer may be caused by several factors. The risk factor that is considered to be the most modifiable is:
    A. gender.
    B. age.
    C. nutrition.
    D. smoking.

14. Which of the following is considered the treatment of choice for early laryngeal cancer?
    A. surgery
    B. chemotherapy
    C. radiation therapy
    D. multiple-drug regimen therapy

15. Your patient is scheduled for a total laryngectomy. Which of the following diagnoses would be the most appropriate to place on the written care plan after the surgery?
    A. Imbalanced Nutrition: Less than Body Requirements
    B. Impaired verbal communication
    C. Anticipatory Grieving
    D. Risk for Aspiration

# CRITICAL THINKING EXERCISE

Read the following situation. Unscramble the words and define each term. Answer the questions using the nursing process of assessment, diagnosis, planning, implementation, and evaluation.

The ambulance team arrived at the emergency room with a patient who had been involved in a fight after a college football game. The patient was slightly combative with slurred speech. An ice pack was placed on the patient's nose during the ride to the hospital. The nurse performed an assessment with the following results: T- 99, P-104, BP-138/76, R-26. Facial *hyccesoism* and *daeem* noted around the nose and eyes. The nasal *petmus* was deviated to the right side. Blood was leaking slowly from the *resan*. The patient's breath smelled of alcohol. The physician's assessment also revealed crepitus. The patient was then diagnosed with a nasal fracture. A simple reduction was performed in the ED, and nasal packing was inserted to control the bleeding. The patient was admitted to the detoxification unit for further evaluation.

1. In addition to the physical assessment, what other information would be important to obtain?
2. Discuss two nursing diagnoses that would be appropriate for this patient. What influence would the alcohol level have on the patient's physical condition?
3. The physician is concerned that the patient may have a CSF leak. What nursing interventions would be initiated at this time to address this problem?
4. Document the patient's condition after the nasal packing was inserted.

# Chapter 24

## Caring for Clients with Lower Respiratory Disorders

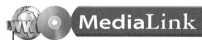
**MediaLink**
**www.prenhall.com/burke**

Use the address above to access the free, interactive Companion Website created for this textbook. Get hints, instant feedback, and textbook references to chapter-related NCLEX-style questions. Link to other interesting sites.

**Audio Glossary:**
Use the Companion Website, or the CD-ROM disk enclosed with your textbook, to hear the pronunciation of key terms in this chapter.

The lower respiratory system is comprised of the bronchi and the lungs. Its function is to allow the exchange of oxygen from the environment and the release of carbon dioxide from the bloodstream. Pathologic problems in any portion of this system prevent the person from experiencing effective oxygenation to the body.

## ANATOMY AND PHYSIOLOGY

Match each term with its appropriate definition.

1. C Barrel chest
2. H Surfactant
3. F Intercostal
4. J Parietal pleura
5. G Left lung

6. E Alveoli
7. D Visceral pleura
8. A Mediastinum

9. B Right lung
10. I Tidal volume

A. Composed of the heart and the great vessels
B. Consists of three lobes
C. Increased anterior-posterior chest diameter
D. Covers the external lung surface
E. Location of oxygen and carbon dioxide exchange
F. Space between the ribs
G. Consists of two lobes
H. Substance that prevents the collapse of the alveoli
I. Amount of air moved with normal breathing
J. Lines the thoracic wall and mediastinum

## FILL IN THE BLANK

Fill in the blanks with the appropriate word or phrase.

1. A technique to improve breathing that incorporates the use of sharply defined exhalations is called ___huff coughing___.

2. The tendency of the lung to return to its original shape and size after exhalation is known as _elasticity_.

3. The condition in which the chest walls float freely due to the fracture of several ribs is referred to as a _flail chest_.

4. A client presents to the clinic with a chronic, nonproductive cough and a history of frequent upper respiratory infections related to cigarette smoking. You anticipate that the physician will diagnose _chronic bronchitis_

5. A type of pneumonia typically seen in the patient with a suppressed immune system, particularly the AIDS patient, is called _pneumocystis carinii_

6. Your patient was found in the supine position with her feeding tube in her hand. Several days later the patient becomes febrile with diminished lung sounds. You suspect that the patient has developed _aspiration pneumonia_

7. A 12-year-old child is brought to the emergency department in respiratory distress. Audible wheezes are noted, along with intercostal muscle retractions. You believe that this client may be suffering from _asthma_.

## MULTIPLE CHOICE

Circle the answer that best completes the following statements.

1. The most common cause of chronic obstructive pulmonary disease is:
   A. environmental pollutants.
   B. alpha-1 antitrypsin deficiency.
   C. heredity.
   D. smoking.

2. A nursing assistant asks you why the lower respiratory system is so important. She understands that you have to breathe in order to live but wants to know the physiology. Your best response would be:
   A. "The lower respiratory tract warms the air."
   B. "The bronchi allow carbon dioxide and oxygen exchange."
   C. "The alveoli produce a substance that helps the lungs move freely."
   D. "Oxygen and carbon dioxide exchange helps to regulate the acid–base balance."

3. The nurse is teaching the client about her asthmatic condition. The focus of the nursing plan should be:
   A. preventing death.
   B. controlling symptoms.
   C. preventing the asthma attack.
   D. instructing about the pathophysiology of asthma as a disease.

4. The client with asthma is being evaluated for ineffective airway clearance. Which of following nursing interventions should be the nurse's highest priority?
   A. Monitor oxygen saturation level.
   B. Check the chart for the latest ABG report.
   C. Assess respiratory effort.
   D. Check the amount and color of sputum.

5. Your patient is complaining of SOB. As you begin your assessment, you note that only the right side of the chest is moving. You next action should be to:
   A. call the charge nurse.
   B. ask the patient why she is only breathing on one side.
   C. apply oxygen at 3 L/nc.
   D. auscultate both lungs.

6. A client was working in a factory that produced a variety of glues. He presents to the emergency room with SOB, fever, and chest pain. Based on your knowledge of pneumonia, you anticipate that this client might have:
   A. aspiration pneumonia.
   B. *Pneumocystis carinii* pneumonia.
   C. tuberculosis.
   D. noninfectious pneumonia.

7. Mr. Jackson will be having a thorocentesis on your shift. If all of the following are appropriate interventions for the client before the procedure, which would have the highest priority?
   A. Tell the client that some pressure will be felt.
   B. Bring the supplies to the bedside.
   C. Administer a cough suppressant, if ordered.
   D. Reinforce teaching about the procedure.

8. The nurse is reading the TB skin test for a client. She measures the redness as 6 mm. This measurement is:
   A. a negative response.
   B. a negative response with no infection.
   C. positive for a person with HIV.
   D. invalid because the induration was not read.

9. Johnny, a 29-year-old HIV patient, has been taking INH for 2 months. He is now complaining of numbness in his feet. You explain that:
   A. this is an unusual side effect.
   B. he needs to be taking vitamin $B_6$ along with the INH.
   C. it is a minor problem and will resolve over time.
   D. it is probably caused by his HIV status.

10. A second-day postoperative client complains of sudden chest pain and SOB. The nurse suspects:
    A. pulmonary embolism.
    B. aspiration pneumonia.
    C. atelectasis.
    D. hemorrhage.

11. You are assessing the chest tube for a patient with lung cancer. You notice that the water in the water seal is fluctuating with the patient's breathing. You next action should be to:
    A. continue with the assessment.
    B. call the physician after your assessment.
    C. ask the patient if he feels okay.
    D. shake the water chamber to stop the bubbling.

12. A 16-year-old male is brought to the emergency room suffering from a severe headache, nausea, and SOB. His skin has a cherry red appearance. You immediately realize that this client may be experiencing:
    A. carbon monoxide poisoning.
    B. status asthmaticus.
    C. walking pneumonia.
    D. cystic fibrosis.

13. During a football game, a player trips and falls. He is brought to the local clinic complaining of severe SOB, tachypnea, and pallor. You note there is asymmetrical lung expansion. You anticipate the insertion of a(n):
    A. IV line.
    B. Foley catheter.
    C. chest tube.
    D. endotracheal tube.

14. The physician has ordered a sputum sample. The nurse knows that the best time to obtain a sputum sample is:
    A. after the first dose of the antibiotic.
    B. right before bedtime.
    C. early in the morning.
    D. late in the afternoon.

15. You are preparing to suction a tracheostomy patient. You remember from your respiratory class that you can apply suction for:
    A. 10 seconds.
    B. 15 seconds.
    C. 25 seconds.
    D. 30 seconds.

## CRITICAL THINKING EXERCISE

Read the following situation. Unscramble the words and define each term. Answer the questions using the nursing process of assessment, diagnosis, planning, implementation, and evaluation.

You are caring for an 18-year-old male client who was admitted for a *eousnotansp mothoneuprax*. His left anterior chest tube was removed yesterday morning. During your assessment you note *spydnea* and decreased breath sounds in the left lung fields. Vital signs: T-100, R-24, P-98, BP-110/68. Thirty minutes later he calls you for help in "breathing." Your focused assessment finds the following: T-100, R-28, P-110, BP-116/72. There are absent lung sounds on the left side, and the trachea is shifted slightly to the right. The client is becoming slightly *noticyac*. The physician diagnoses a *sionten pneuthoraxmo*.

1. During the focused assessment, what action should the nurse take after noting the absent breath sounds?
2. Based on the client's diagnosis, what can you anticipate will be ordered?
3. List five items to be assessed after the procedure.
4. Name one nursing diagnosis that should be included on the care plan.

# Chapter 25

# The Cardiovascular System and Assessment

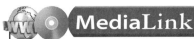
The heart, blood, and blood vessels, collectively known as the cardiovascular system, work together as a fuel delivery and waste removal system for the body. The heart, a simple pump, pushes blood through a system of blood vessels to deliver oxygen and glucose to the cells and tissues. Focused assessment of the client with cardiovascular disease begins by asking about current symptoms.

## ANATOMY AND PHYSIOLOGY

Match each term with its appropriate definition.

1. _A_ Sternum
2. _E_ Pericardium
3. _F_ Superior vena cava
4. _I_ Pulmonary artery
5. _C_ Coronary arteries
6. _G_ Sinoatrial node
7. _J_ Purkinje fibers
8. _H_ Depolarization
9. _D_ Internodal pathways
10. _B_ Tricuspid valve

A. Plate of bone forming the middle of the thorax

B. Flap of tissue between the right atrium and ventricle

C. Supplies oxygen and nutrients to the cardiac muscle

D. Means for electrical currents to pass between nodes

E. Sac surrounding the heart and base of great vessels

F. Transports deoxygenated blood from upper body

G. Pacemaker of the heart

H. Reversal of positive and negative charges

I. Carries deoxygenated blood from the right ventricle

J. Forms the last part of the heart conduction system

# FILL IN THE BLANK

Fill in the blanks with the appropriate word or phrase.

1.  The heart, a hollow, cone-shaped organ approximately the size of an adult's fist, weighs _less than 1 lb_.

2.  The heart is covered by the *pericardium*. The pericardium encases the heart and anchors it to surrounding structures. It has two layers: the _parietal_ and the _visceral_ pericardium.

3.  The _cardiac tendons_ prevent the backflow of blood during contraction of the higher pressure ventricles.

4.  Unlike skeletal muscle tissue, _cardiac_ can generate an electrical impulse and contraction independent of the nervous system.

5.  The action potential generated by pacemaker cells is caused by the movement of _ions_ across cell membranes.

6.  With each contraction, _stroke volume_ causes approximately 70 mL of blood (in an adult) to be ejected from the heart.

7.  _Cardiac reserve_ is the ability of the heart to increase cardiac output and blood pressure to meet the demand.

# MULTIPLE CHOICE

Circle the answer that best completes the following statements.

1.  The AV valves close as the ventricles start to contract, producing the first heart sound called:
    A.  $S_1$.
    B.  $S_2$.
    C.  $S_3$.
    D.  $S_4$.

2.  The heartbeat is controlled by specialized cells within the myocardium known as the:
    A.  nervous system.
    B.  respiratory system.
    C.  conduction system.
    D.  cardiac system.

3.  The sinoatrial (SA) node usually generates an impulse:
    A.  40 to 60 times per minute.
    B.  50 times per minute.
    C.  60 to 100 times per minute.
    D.  100 times per minute.

4.  The action potential and depolarization cause muscle to:
    A.  beat.
    B.  contract.
    C.  twitch.
    D.  elevate.

5. Ventricular filling occurs when the ventricles are relaxed during:
   A. systole.
   B. heartbeat.
   C. contraction.
   D. diastole.

6. Arteries, veins, and capillaries are included in the:
   A. cardiac system.
   B. GI system.
   C. peripheral vascular system.
   D. pulmonary system.

7. A noninvasive test that has been shown to be highly indicative of atherosclerosis is called a(n):
   A. ankle-brachial index.
   B. ECG.
   C. femoral-cephalic index.
   D. Holter monitor.

8. These hormones are released by the heart muscle in response to changes in blood volume.
   A. ANF
   B. estrogen
   C. BMP
   D. testosterone

9. Stress testing is used to detect asymptomatic coronary heart disease and may cause:
   A. an increase in pulse rate.
   B. exhaustion.
   C. an increase in stress.
   D. a cardiac emergency.

10. A transthoracic echocardiogram (TTE) is:
    A. expensive.
    B. dangerous.
    C. invasive.
    D. noninvasive.

## CRITICAL THINKING EXERCISE

Read the following situation. Unscramble the words and define each term. Answer the questions using the nursing process of assessment, diagnosis, planning, implementation, and evaluation.

The *doimgraceeltcro* is a record of the heart's electrical activity detected by electrodes placed on the skin. ECG waveforms and patterns are used to detect *tmssyydrhiah, ymlaaroicd* damage or enlargement, and the effects of drugs. Electrocardiography may be used on a *intlaunoc* or *tetnttremiin* basis, depending on the client's needs.

1. What other diagnostic tests are used to detect cardiac disorders?

2. What signs and symptoms might the nurse observe in a patient with abnormalities?

3. Name three possible nursing diagnoses for a patient with cardiac disorders.

# Chapter 26

## Caring for Clients with Coronary Heart Disease and Dysrhythmias

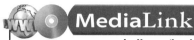

**www.prenhall.com/burke**

Use the address above to access the free, interactive Companion Website created for this textbook. Get hints, instant feedback, and textbook references to chapter-related NCLEX-style questions. Link to other interesting sites.

**Audio Glossary:**

Use the Companion Website, or the CD-ROM disk enclosed with your textbook, to hear the pronunciation of key terms in this chapter.

Cardiovascular disease (CVD) is the leading cause of death and disability in the United States. Approximately 21 million people are affected by heart disease and more than 700,000 people die from it each year. Nurses need to know about heart disease and its causes to teach and effectively care for clients with coronary heart disease and dysrhythmias.

## CORONARY ARTERY DISEASE

Match each term with its appropriate definition.

1. _____ CAD
2. _____ Atherosclerosis
3. _____ Angina pectoris
4. _____ Sedentary
5. _____ Metabolic syndrome
6. _____ Homocysteine
7. _____ Ischemic
8. _____ Myalgias
9. _____ Prinzmetal's
10. _____ Cardiogenic shock

A. Physical inactivity
B. An amino acid linked to CAD
C. Impaired blood flow to the heart muscle
D. Muscle aches
E. A group of related risk factors occurring in the same person
F. Without enough blood and oxygen to meet metabolic needs
G. A narrowing of the coronary arteries due plaque formation
H. Impaired tissue perfusion due to pump failure
I. Episodic chest pain
J. A typical angina that occurs without an identified precipitating cause, often waking the client from sleep

## FILL IN THE BLANK

Fill in the blanks with the appropriate word or phrase.

1. Beth Anne, 36, comes into the clinic complaining of shortness of breath, nausea, and jaw pain. Based on her symptoms, you suspect _____.

2. An MI usually attacks the _____ because of its larger muscle mass and increased oxygen demands.

3. An arteriogram shows numerous plaque formations in a client's abdominal aorta. The disease that most likely will result from these substances is called _____.

4. Mr. Stevenson reports that he has been waking up at night because of pain in his chest. The most likely type of angina that will be diagnosed is _____.

5. The nurse is explaining to a client that the surgeon will use a balloon-tipped catheter to increase the blood flow in an occluded artery. This procedure is called _____.

6. A 48-year-old male arrives in the emergency room complaining of severe pain in his chest. He is pale and diaphoretic. He tells the nurse that he feels as if he might die. This client is most likely experiencing a _____.

7. You are assessing a client, 72, who has the following signs and symptoms: episodes of dizziness, light-headedness, fainting, palpitations, chest pain, or shortness of breath. You anticipate that the physician will diagnose this client with _____.

## MULTIPLE CHOICE

Circle the answer that best completes the following statements.

1. The nurse is explaining the purpose of an electrocardiogram to a group of nursing students. The nurse would be correct if she said:
   A. "It allows the doctor to view the inside of the heart."
   B. "It produces a picture of the electrical activity of the heart."
   C. "It is used to increase the diameter of the artery."
   D. "It is a device that temporarily takes over the function of the SA node."

2. If all of the following are true, which assessment data should be the highest priority for the nurse to obtain from the client with a dysrhythmia?
   A. History of falls
   B. Smoking habits
   C. History of cardiovascular disease
   D. Current medications

3. A client has received instructions on his new pacemaker. Which of these comments, if made by the client, indicates a need for further teaching?
   A. "I'll carry my pacemaker card in my wallet."
   B. "If my pulse drops lower than the set rate, I'll take a rest break."
   C. "I will call the doctor if I have any chest pain."
   D. "I should see my doctor on a regular schedule."

4. You are walking in the parking lot at the grocery store when you see a woman lying by her car. Your next action should be:
   A. call for help.
   B. begin CPR.
   C. ask the woman if she is okay.
   D. check for a pulse.

5. A client presents to the clinic with complaints of orthopnea and severe pedal edema. He tells the nurse that he is taking Lasix and digoxin for congestive heart failure. The assessment reveals an elevated BP, crackles throughout the lung fields and 3+ pitting edema. The most appropriate nursing diagnosis would be:
   A. Noncompliance.
   B. Tissue Perfusion, Ineffective (Cardiopulmonary).
   C. Risk of Skin Impairment.
   D. Fluid Volume Excess.

6. Several hours after a client has returned from a coronary angiography, you notice that the dressing is saturated with blood. Your next action should be to:
   A. call the doctor.
   B. check for a pulse distal to the incision.
   C. reinforce the dressing.
   D. apply pressure to the site.

7. Which of the following would not be discussed with a patient scheduled for cardiac surgery?
   A. coughing and deep breathing exercises
   B. special cardiac diet prior to the surgery
   C. visiting hours after the surgery
   D. proper use of antiembolic hose

8. A client asks you if his cholesterol level of 210 is within the normal range. Your response should be:
   A. "It all depends on which level you are talking about, the total or the LDL."
   B. "That is high. It should be under 200."
   C. "You have to ask your doctor about that."
   D. "I'm not sure. Let me go check my lab reference book."

9. A client is to receive a morning dose of digoxin. Which finding, if present, would indicate that the medication should not be given?
   A. radial pulse of 80
   B. apical pulse of 52
   C. radial pulse of 60
   D. apical pulse of 62

10. A client with a history of rheumatic heart disease has been scheduled for a tooth extraction. Which of the following would the nurse anticipate the dentist will prescribe for this client before the procedure?
    A. anticoagulant
    B. antibiotic
    C. cardiotonic
    D. ACE inhibitor

## CRITICAL THINKING EXERCISE

Read the following situation. Unscramble the words and define each term. Answer the questions using the nursing process of assessment, diagnosis, planning, implementation, and evaluation.

The *rhaet* contracts in response to electrical stimulation of its cells. In the normal heart, this produces a coordinated, rhythmic contraction that pushes blood into *tlccauirino*. The normal heart rhythm is normal sinus rhythm (NSR). Impulses originate in the *oirlatrasn* (SA or sinus) node and travel through normal conduction pathways without delay. The rate is between 60 and 100 bpm. Changes from this rhythm can affect the heart's ability to pump blood effectively to body tissues.

1. What is a cardiac dysrhythmia? How does it occur and how do you treat it?
2. What is the suggested sequence of steps in interpreting an ECG strip?
3. Cardiac rhythms are classified according to the site of impulse formation or the site and degree of conduction block. Name and define at least three rhythms.

# Chapter 27

# Caring for Clients with Cardiac Disorders

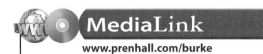

**www.prenhall.com/burke**

Use the address above to access the free, interactive Companion Website created for this textbook. Get hints, instant feedback, and textbook references to chapter-related NCLEX-style questions. Link to other interesting sites.

**Audio Glossary:**

Use the Companion Website, or the CD-ROM disk enclosed with your textbook, to hear the pronunciation of key terms in this chapter.

Disorders of the heart muscle or its structures affect its ability to effectively pump blood to meet the needs of the cells of the body. When the heart is unable to function effectively, other organ systems may fail because their fuel supply is impaired.

## ANATOMY AND PHYSIOLOGY

Match each term with its appropriate definition.

1. _____ Heart failure

2. _____ Ventricular hypertrophy

3. _____ Cardiac reserve

4. _____ Orthopnea

5. _____ Pulmonary edema

6. _____ PND

7. _____ Inotropic

8. _____ Cardiomyoplasty

9. _____ Rheumatic fever

10. _____ Endocarditis

A. Wrapping a skeletal muscle graft around the heart to lend support to the failing myocardium

B. Breathing difficulty while lying down

C. Condition in which the client awakens at night acutely short of breath

D. An infectious process that usually affects clients with underlying heart disease

E. Enlarged cardiac muscle cells

F. Drugs that increase the strength of the heart's contractions

G. Allows the heart to adjust its output to meet the metabolic needs of the body

H. A systemic inflammatory disease caused by an abnormal immune response to infection by group A beta-hemolytic streptococci

I. The inability of the heart to function as a pump to meet the needs of the body

J. Accumulation of fluid in the interstitial spaces and alveoli of the lungs

## FILL IN THE BLANK

Fill in the blanks with the appropriate word or phrase.

1. Organisms in the bloodstream attach to the endocardial lining of the heart and become enmeshed in deposits of fibrin and platelets. This covering "protects" the bacteria from quick removal by the immune system. These vegetations develop on heart valve leaflets, varying in size and shape and are easily _____ breaking off and traveling through the bloodstream to other organs.

2. _____ is an inflammatory disorder of the heart muscle that may be caused by infection (viral, bacterial, and protozoal), an immune response, radiation, chemical poisons, drugs, or burns.

3. Ms. Parson's, age 45, with end-stage kidney disease, has developed chest pain relieved by sitting up and leaning forward, and a fever of 102. You suspect she may have _____ when you hear a friction rub on auscultation of her heart.

4. Mitch, 42, is status post-CABG. You are taking his vital signs when you notice that his systolic blood pressure drops more than 10 mm Hg during inspiration. You recognize this as a _____.

5. The nurse recognizes the above situation with Mitch as a medical emergency called _____.

6. _____ may be done as an emergency procedure for cardiac tamponade. The physician inserts a large (16- to 18-gauge) needle into the pericardial sac and withdraws excess fluid.

7. You are assessing a client who has the following signs and symptoms: distended jugular veins, edema in the sacrum and lower extremities, nausea. You anticipate that the physician will diagnose this client with _____.

## MULTIPLE CHOICE

Circle the answer that best completes the following statements.

1. You are instructing a nursing student in the correct administration of a nitroglycerin patch. The most important point that should be made at this time is to:
   A. wipe off the old medication before applying the new patch.
   B. rotate sites.
   C. wear gloves.
   D. not massage into the skin.

2. A client has been admitted to the hospital in acute heart failure. Which of the following diets would the nurse expect to see ordered for the patient?
   A. low-fat, high-protein
   B. high-potassium, low-protein
   C. low-sodium, high-protein
   D. high-protein, high-sodium

3.  Which of the following nursing diagnoses would be most appropriate for the client in congestive heart failure?
    A.  Activity intolerance
    B.  Knowledge Deficit
    C.  Pain, Acute
    D.  Deficient Fluid Volume

4.  A client in end-stage renal disease has been diagnosed with pericarditis. Which intervention would the nurse expect to include in the nursing care plan?
    A.  assist with a pericardiocentesis
    B.  administer NSAIDS
    C.  assess the lung sounds every 8 hours
    D.  place the bed in low-Fowler's position

5.  A 28-year-old female, pregnant with her second child, arrives in the emergency room with severe SOB and hemoptysis. The physician tells you that the client's lungs are "wet" and that he is able to detect a diastolic murmur. You suspect that this client has:
    A.  aspiration pneumonia.
    B.  pulmonary edema.
    C.  right-sided heart failure.
    D.  cardiac tamponade.

6.  Valvular heart disease interferes with blood flow to and from the heart. The most common cause of this disease is:
    A.  pericarditis.
    B.  MI.
    C.  CHF.
    D.  rheumatic fever.

7.  Valve disorders affect pressures and blood flow both in front of and behind the affected valve. The two major types of heart valve disorders are:
    A.  aspiration and pneumonia.
    B.  pulmonic and edema.
    C.  stenosis and regurgitation.
    D.  cardiac and pulmonic.

8.  Jane, a 28-year-old female, pregnant with her first child, arrives in the emergency room with severe SOB, fatigue, and palpitations. The physician tells you that he is able to detect a diastolic murmur. You suspect that this client has:
    A.  mitral regurgitation.
    B.  mitral stenosis.
    C.  right-sided heart failure.
    D.  cardiac tamponade.

9.  You are assessing your client and hear a "seagull-like" murmur at the apex of his heart. You suspect that this client has:
    A.  mitral regurgitation.
    B.  mitral stenosis.
    C.  right-sided heart failure.
    D.  cardiac tamponade.

10. Marty, 56, came in with angina, dyspnea, and syncope. His prognosis is grim; most clients get progressively worse and die within 2 years of the onset of symptoms. You suspect that this client has:
    A. cardiac tamponade.
    B. myocarditis.
    C. cardiomyopathy.
    D. pericarditis.

## CRITICAL THINKING EXERCISE

Read the following situation. Unscramble the words and define each term. Answer the questions using the nursing process of assessment, diagnosis, planning, implementation, and evaluation.

Endocarditis, inflammation of the *ucndaredmoi,* is an infectious process that usually affects clients with underlying heart disease. *Tabcraie* often enter through invasive procedures or devices, such as intravenous catheters, indwelling urinary catheters, dental procedures, or during heart surgery. The left side of the heart, the *tmrila* valve in particular, is the most common site of infection. *Vtinnuosare* drug use is also a risk factor; in these individuals, the right side (the *dtiirucsp* valve) is often involved.

1. Discuss the classification and onset of endocarditis.
2. Discuss the physical manifestations of endocarditis.
3. Discuss the pathophysiology of this diagnosis.

# Chapter 28

## Caring for Clients with Peripheral Vascular Disorders

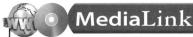
**MediaLink**
www.prenhall.com/burke

Use the address above to access the free, interactive Companion Website created for this textbook. Get hints, instant feedback, and textbook references to chapter-related NCLEX-style questions. Link to other interesting sites.

**Audio Glossary:**
Use the Companion Website, or the CD-ROM disk enclosed with your textbook, to hear the pronunciation of key terms in this chapter.

The peripheral vascular system includes all arteries and veins that are distal to the heart. Disrupted or diminished flow of blood to any part of the body can lead to pain and fatal tissue necrosis. The nursing care focuses on assisting the client in the prevention of these disorders and in the relief of the physical and emotional pain that accompanies each.

## ANATOMY AND PHYSIOLOGY

Match each term with its appropriate definition.

1. _____ Capillary
2. _____ Tunica adventitia
3. _____ Valves
4. _____ Tunica media
5. _____ Tunica intima
6. _____ Arterioles
7. _____ Baroreceptors
8. _____ Viscosity
9. _____ PVR
10. _____ Chemoreceptors

A. Inner layer of vessel wall
B. Special cells that are sensitive to chemicals
C. Middle layer of vessel containing smooth muscle
D. Located in vessels to prevent backflow of blood
E. Minute vessel that connects arterioles and venules
F. Protects and anchors vessels
G. Thickness of a substance
H. Cells that are sensitive to blood pressure changes
I. Tiny arterial branch
J. Opposing forces to blood flow

## FILL IN THE BLANK

Fill in the blanks with the appropriate word or phrase.

1. An African American male presents to the clinic with a blood pressure of 190/120. His medical history includes hypokalemia, obesity, and chronic bronchitis. The physician diagnoses this client with _____.

2. A 210-pound male, age 42, is admitted to the ICU with a blood pressure of 220/140. He is confused and complains of a severe headache. The nurse recognizes this emergency as _____.

3. A client tells the nurse that he is unable to walk more than 15 feet without having severe pain in the calves of his legs. The pain goes away when resting. This client most likely will be diagnosed as having _____.

4. A 32-year-old male is seen in your clinic with a cramping pain in his foot. His toes are pale and cool to the touch, and the nails are thick. He tells you that he has been smoking most of his life. You anticipate that the physician will diagnose this client with _____.

5. A young woman reports that her fingers turn blue and red during the winter months. She states that there is some numbness and occasional pain during these episodes. The nurse is aware that these signs and symptoms may indicate _____.

6. An elderly client is transported to the emergency room by the paramedics. Upon arrival, the client complains of severe pain in his lower back. Inspection reveals a pulsating mass in the upper abdomen. The nurse suspects that this client has an _____.

7. A postoperative patient has been on bed rest for 3 days. He tells you that his right calf is swollen, red, and tender. You expect that this patient has developed _____.

## MULTIPLE CHOICE

Circle the answer that best completes the following statements.

1. Mr. Greggs, age 68, is being seen in the clinic for a routine physical. He is of Jewish ancestry. He tells you that he smokes a half-pack of cigarettes per day and enjoys popcorn and sodas as a snack. His weight is 205 pounds. Which of these risk factors is considered unalterable in the prevention of hypertension?
   A. family history
   B. smoking
   C. high sodium intake
   D. obesity

2. The nurse is teaching the assistant how to take a blood pressure. Further teaching is indicated if the assistant:
   A. centers the cuff directly over the artery.
   B. palpates the artery before beginning the procedure.
   C. inflates the cuff 80 mm Hg over the pulse level.
   D. chooses the cuff at 40% arm circumference.

3. Which of the following should be included on a nursing care plan for a patient with peripheral vascular disease?
   A. Dry the feet carefully by rubbing briskly.
   B. Buy shoes in the morning before swelling begins.
   C. Check the temperature of the water before stepping into the tub.
   D. Do not use powder on the feet.

4. You are caring for a patient who has had aortic surgery. You know to assess for signs of graft leakage. If all of the following are true, which would be considered the highest priority for nursing intervention?
   A. hematoma at the incision
   B. decreasing peripheral pulses
   C. increased abdominal girth
   D. decreasing blood pressure

5. The nurse is preparing a care plan for a patient with DVT. All of the following nursing diagnoses are appropriate except:
   A. Pain, Acute
   B. Ineffective Peripheral Tissue Perfusion
   C. Impaired Skin Integrity
   D. Risk for Constipation

6. A client, diagnosed with HTN, has been started on an ACE inhibitor. You know that the action of this medication to reduce blood pressure is due to:
   A. the blocking of the sympathetic input to the heart.
   B. inhibition of the renin–angiotensin–aldosterone mechanism.
   C. the slowing of the heart rate by reducing vasoconstriction.
   D. the relaxation of vascular smooth muscle.

7. Your client has a blood pressure of 164/100. You anticipate that the physician will:
   A. recheck the BP in 1 year.
   B. confirm the BP within 2 months.
   C. refer for evaluation within 1 month.
   D. refer for evaluation within 1 week.

8. You are teaching a client about a diet low in vitamin K. You know that the client understands the instructions by telling you that:
   A. "I will buy boxed macaroni and cheese instead of making it from scratch."
   B. "I will eat lots of yogurt because I need the calcium."
   C. "I will buy 1% milk from now on."
   D. "I will stop buying spinach for a few months."

9. A 46-year-old executive asks you to help him understand how to reduce the stress in his life. He has recently been diagnosed with primary hypertension. Your best response should be:
   A. "Stop worrying about everything."
   B. "Exercise regularly everyday."
   C. "Take a class that focuses on therapeutic touch."
   D. "Join a meditation group."

10. The primary manifestation of peripheral arterial disease is:
    A. pain.
    B. dependent rubor.
    C. intermittent claudication.
    D. decreased pulses.

11. A patient with DVT suddenly develops chest pain and SOB. The nurse suspects that this patient has developed:
    A. an embolism.
    B. atelectasis.
    C. spontaneous pneumothorax.
    D. bacterial pneumonia.

12. During the physical assessment, the nurse discovers that there are no palpable pedal pulses in the client's left foot. Her next action should be to:
    A. reattempt to palpate the pulses.
    B. ask the charge nurse to palpate the pulses.
    C. obtain a Doppler.
    D. document the absent pulses.

13. A patient has been diagnosed with severe peripheral vascular disease. The nurse anticipates that the physician will order a low dose of aspirin. The rationale for the use of this medication is that:
    A. aspirin decreases the risk for clot formation.
    B. aspirin is an analgesic.
    C. aspirin can prevent a fever from occurring.
    D. aspirin is contraindicated in the patient with PVD.

14. You are discussing nursing interventions with the charge nurse for a patient with PVD. You suggest that the following intervention should be included:
    A. Gatch the knee at a 90-degree angle.
    B. Instruct the client to keep the extremity in an independent position.
    C. Use a heating pad to keep the extremity warm.
    D. Assess the peripheral pulses every 4 hours.

15. The physician has prescribed the drug Coumadin for a patient with arterial disease. Which of the following should be included in the patient teaching?
    A. Increase the amount of vitamin K in the diet.
    B. Report any unusual bruises.
    C. Have blood levels of the medication taken every 6 months.
    D. Double the dose of the medication if a dose is skipped.

## CRITICAL THINKING EXERCISE

Read the following situation. Unscramble the words and define each term. Answer the questions use the nursing process of assessment, diagnosis, planning, implementation, and evaluation.

A 46-year-old female presents to your clinic with complaints of severe, aching leg pain, along with a feeling of "heavy" legs. She tells you that she has been a nurse for more than 20 years. Inspection of the legs shows tortuous vessels in the great *ehpassonu* vein and brown skin discolorations above the ankle.

The physician orders a *pperdol sonicultra owlf estt* and some *ggphicaanrio* studies. The results of these tests indicate that this client is a candidate for *neiv ppiingtrs*.

1. Based on the data, what type of PVD is this client experiencing?
2. What factors contributed to the development of this diagnosis?
3. Name one major complication that may result from this problem.
4. Document three nursing interventions for the diagnosis of Ineffective Tissue Perfusion.

# Chapter 29

# The Hematologic and Lymphatic Systems and Assessment

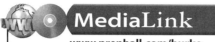

**MediaLink**

**www.prenhall.com/burke**

Use the address above to access the free, interactive Companion Website created for this textbook. Get hints, instant feedback, and textbook references to chapter-related NCLEX-style questions. Link to other interesting sites.

**Audio Glossary:**

Use the Companion Website, or the CD-ROM disk enclosed with your textbook, to hear the pronunciation of key terms in this chapter.

Nurses play an important role in identifying many of the manifestations of hematologic and lymphatic system disorders. Assessment of these systems generally is conducted as part of the general survey of the client's health or concurrently with focused cardiovascular system assessment.

## HEMATOLOGIC TERMS

Match each term with its appropriate definition.

| | |
|---|---|
| 1. _____ Plasma | A. An essential part of the body's clotting mechanism |
| 2. _____ Stem Cells | B. Hormone that stimulates the bone marrow to produce RBCs |
| 3. _____ Erythrocytes | C. A clear yellow, protein-rich fluid |
| 4. _____ Erythropoietin | D. An oxygen-carrying protein |
| 5. _____ Hemoglobin | E. Part of the body's defense against infection and disease |
| 6. _____ Hemolysis | F. The beginning of all cells |
| 7. _____ Transferrin | G. Shaped like *biconcave disks* |
| 8. _____ Leukocytes | H. Iron that circulates in the bloodstream |
| 9. _____ Phagocytes | I. Responsible for engulfing and destroying foreign matter |
| 10. _____ Platelets | J. The process of RBC destruction |

# FILL IN THE BLANK

Fill in the blanks with the appropriate word or phrase.

1. Platelets live approximately _____ in circulating blood.

2. The five stages in hemostasis are _____, _____, _____, _____, _____.

3. The lymphatic system has several functions: _____, _____, and _____.

4. Assessment of the hematologic and lymphatic systems begins with inspection of the color of the skin and mucous membranes for _____ or _____.

5. The nurse knows that a _____ is often performed as a routine screening examination and may include a hemoglobin and hematocrit level.

6. Mr. Burke is hospitalized for cardiovascular disease. He is scheduled for CABG in the morning. The nurse knows an important lab that will be ordered prior to surgery is _____.

7. A _____ is used to diagnose aplastic anemia, leukemias, and other cancers.

# MULTIPLE CHOICE

Circle the answer that best completes the following statements.

1. A laboratory test used to diagnose hemolytic anemias and investigate transfusion reactions is called:
   A. electrophoresis.
   B. coagulation.
   C. Coombs'.
   D. Schilling's.

2. Before a bone marrow aspiration, the nurse should have the client:
   A. maintain a full bladder.
   B. in reverse Trendelenburg position.
   C. sign consent.
   D. cough.

3. A patient is undergoing a biopsy to rule out malignancy of her left supra-clavicular lymph node. The nurse tells her prior to the procedure:
   A. "You can't eat for 24 hours after the procedure."
   B. "You will bleed excessively following the procedure."
   C. "You are only allowed two visitors every thirty minutes."
   D. "I will monitor your vital signs routinely after the procedure."

4. The primary function of RBCs is to:
   A. transport oxygen to the cells.
   B. provide immunity to the body.
   C. destroy foreign matter.
   D. control bleeding.

5. Mr. Kelp is diagnosed with iron-deficiency anemia. You should recommend a diet of increased:
   A. organ meats.
   B. fruits.
   C. bread.
   D. dairy products.

6. A Schilling test is used to diagnose:
   A. addiction.
   B. pernicious anemia.
   C. aplastic anemia.
   D. cancer.

7. Mary, 11, was diagnosed with leukemia. The nurse knows to watch for what observation in her assessment?
   A. scales and rashes
   B. petechiae and purpura
   C. bowel and bladder control
   D. loss of sensation

8. The most serious hazard for a patient who has had a bone marrow aspiration is:
   A. hemorrhage.
   B. pain.
   C. bruising.
   D. shock.

9. Evaluates the extrinsic clotting pathway; prolonged in Coumadin therapy:
   A. INR.
   B. PTT.
   C. PT.
   D. APTT.

10. A 28-year-old patient's transferrin lab has come back slightly elevated. You ask her if she is taking:
    A. cocaine.
    B. amphetamines.
    C. Coumadin.
    D. oral contraceptives.

## CRITICAL THINKING EXERCISE

Read the following situation. Unscramble the words and define each term. Answer the questions using the nursing process of assessment, diagnosis, planning, implementation, and evaluation.

Blood transports *xnoyge* and *ttiennsur* to cells, essential *sstbunaces* (such as hormones and other chemical messengers) to *lelcs* and tissues, and *swtae* products away from tissues for removal from the body.

1. What are some other terms associated with red blood cells?
2. Granulocytes are the most plentiful of white blood cells. What is their percentage of total leukocytes? Name the different types of granulocytes.
3. Discuss the role of lymphocytes in the body.

# Chapter 30

## Caring for Clients with Hematologic and Lymphatic Disorders

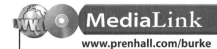

**www.prenhall.com/burke**

Use the address above to access the free, interactive Companion Website created for this textbook. Get hints, instant feedback, and textbook references to chapter-related NCLEX-style questions. Link to other interesting sites.

**Audio Glossary:**

Use the Companion Website, or the CD-ROM disk enclosed with your textbook, to hear the pronunciation of key terms in this chapter.

Disorders affecting the red blood cells affect the body's ability to carry oxygen to the tissues. As a result, the client often experiences manifestations such as fatigue and activity intolerance. Care for clients with lymphatic system disorders focuses on relieving edema, maintaining skin integrity in the affected extremity, and preventing or treating infection.

## ANATOMY AND PHYSIOLOGY

Match each term with its appropriate definition.

1. _____ Anemia
2. _____ Polycythemia
3. _____ Myeloma
4. _____ Leukemia
5. _____ Agranulocytosis
6. _____ Hemophilia
7. _____ DIC
8. _____ Lymphangitis
9. _____ Malignant lymphoma
10. _____ Thrombocytopenia

A. A complex disorder characterized by simultaneous blood clotting and hemorrhages

B. A group of malignant disorders of WBCs

C. Hemoglobin concentration or the number of circulating RBCs is decreased

D. A group of hereditary clotting factor deficiencies

E. A platelet count of less than 100,000 platelets per milliliter of blood

F. Characterized by lymphocyte proliferation

G. A decrease in granulocytes

H. Excess erythropoietin production

I. Malignancy in which plasma cells multiply uncontrollably and infiltrate bone marrow, lymph nodes, and other tissues

J. Inflammation of the lymph vessels

# FILL IN THE BLANK

Fill in the blanks with the appropriate word or phrase.

1. A 34-year-old man complains of abdominal pain with a 1-week history. The client is in your clinic because he is concerned about the continuous pain. His hemoglobin is 9 g/dL. You suspect the client is experiencing a(n) _____.

2. A 20-year-old woman has presented in your clinic for complaints of a sore throat and fatigue. Vital signs are T-102, BP-124/82, P-96, and R-20. On palpation of her neck, you note swollen lymph nodes. You also note enlargement of the spleen. The physician orders a WBC count and throat culture. The lab results indicate elevated WBCs. Based on these findings you understand the client has mononucleosis caused by the _____virus.

3. _____ is more common than Hodgkin's disease.

4. The diagnosis of lymphoma is made based on biopsy of tissue from the enlarged node or tissue mass. If _____ cells are present, the diagnosis of Hodgkin's disease is confirmed.

5. _____ results in complete remission in more than 75% of clients with Hodgkin's disease who do not have systemic symptoms.

6. _____ and _____ (symptoms of lymphoma) increase the risk for skin lesions.

7. _____, lack of RBCs and hemoglobin, is a common disorder.

# MULTIPLE CHOICE

Circle the answer that best completes the following statements.

1. Acquired hemolytic anemia results when RBCs are damaged by outside factors, such as:
   A. immune responses.
   B. cellular.
   C. healing.
   D. stress.

2. Aplastic anemia may follow injury to stem cells in bone marrow caused by:
   A. certain infections.
   B. drugs or radiation.
   C. chemicals.
   D. all of the above.

3. Aplastic anemia if left untreated could ultimately lead to:
   A. leukocytosis.
   B. leukopenia.
   C. nothing; it corrects itself.
   D. heart failure.

4. Sickle cell anemia usually affects people of:
   A. Mediterranean descent.
   B. Asian descent.
   C. African descent.
   D. European descent.

5. Myelodysplastic syndrome (MDS) is a group of stem cell disorders characterized by abnormal appearing bone marrow and ineffective blood cell production. It is primarily a disorder of:
   A. middle adults.
   B. young adults.
   C. older adults.
   D. children.

6. After an autologous bone marrow transplant, the risk of death is greater for a patient due to:
   A. microorganisms.
   B. bleeding.
   C. immunosuppression.
   D. pain.

7. An alternative to bone marrow transplant is:
   A. brain cell transplant.
   B. stem cell transplant.
   C. spinal fluid transplant.
   D. all of the above.

8. The inheritance patterns for both hemophilia A and B are:
   A. Y-linked recessive disorders.
   B. X-linked recessive disorders.
   C. female reproductive disorders.
   D. male reproductive disorders.

9. A person with Hodgkin's may have a nursing diagnosis of:
   A. Risk for impaired skin integrity.
   B. Disturbed thought processes.
   C. Deficient Fluid volume.
   D. None of the above.

10. Exposure to environmental toxins such as radiation and benzene and cancer treatment with radiation and chemotherapy are identified risk factors for:
    A. AIDS.
    B. BMT.
    C. SCT.
    D. MDS.

## CRITICAL THINKING EXERCISE

Read the following situation. Unscramble the words and define each term. Answer the questions using the nursing process of assessment, diagnosis, planning, implementation, and evaluation.

Nursing care of the client with *lmaignnat* lymphoma involves providing physical and emotional *ppusrot* throughout the course of treatment. The client is at risk for *ftniiecon* because cancerous *ptymlhoyctse* are less effective in mounting an immune response. *Lnttriinuao* status also must be considered due to the effects of the disease and treatment on appetite and food tolerance.

1. In addition to the physical assessment, what other information would be important to obtain?

2. Discuss three nursing diagnoses that would be appropriate for this client.

3. What is the treatment most likely to be prescribed and what are the nursing implications?

# Chapter 31

# The Urinary System and Assessment

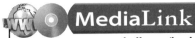

**www.prenhall.com/burke**

Use the address above to access the free, interactive Companion Website created for this textbook. Get hints, instant feedback, and textbook references to chapter-related NCLEX-style questions. Link to other interesting sites.

**Audio Glossary:**

Use the Companion Website, or the CD-ROM disk enclosed with your textbook, to hear the pronunciation of key terms in this chapter.

The urinary system plays a vital role in eliminating wastes and regulating fluid and electrolyte balance in the body. Changes in its structure or function can affect the entire body; likewise, it is affected by other body systems, particularly the cardio-vascular and endocrine systems.

## ANATOMY AND PHYSIOLOGY

Match each term with its appropriate definition.

| | |
|---|---|
| 1. _____ Glomeruli | A. Chief end product of protein metabolism |
| 2. _____ Nephrons | B. Formed in muscle and excreted in the urine |
| 3. _____ Ureter | C. Functional units of the kidney |
| 4. _____ Urinary meatus | D. Small clusters of capillaries |
| 5. _____ GFR | E. Rate at which blood is filtered in the glomeruli |
| 6. _____ Urethra | F. Moves urine from the kidneys to the bladder by peristaltic waves |
| 7. _____ Proximal tubules | G. Small channels that begin the filtration process |
| 8. _____ Renin | H. Opening of urinary path to the outside of the body |
| 9. _____ Urea | I. Tube that carries urine outside of the body |
| 10. _____ Creatinine | J. Plays a role in the regulation of blood pressure |

# FILL IN THE BLANK

Fill in the blanks with the appropriate word or phrase.

1. Healthy adults usually feel the urge to void when the bladder contains _____ mL of urine.

2. In males, the _____ is about 8 inches (20 cm) long; it serves as a channel for semen as well as urine.

3. A drop in _____ or blood volume causes the GFR and urine output to fall.

4. Urine is composed, by volume, of about _____ water and _____ solutes.

5. The kidneys are less able to concentrate urine in the older adult. This fact, combined with diminished thirst in older adults, increases the risk for _____.

6. Jon comes into the clinic complaining of cloudy, foul-smelling urine. The nurse knows this is called _____.

7. Before a diagnosis can be made on a client's urinary status, the nurse knows that a _____ must be obtained and that the urine should be inspected for color, odor, and clarity before being sent to the laboratory.

# MULTIPLE CHOICE

Circle the answer that best completes the following statements.

1. Your patient has been ordered to have a post-void residual catheterization. Which of the following statements made by the patient indicates understanding of the procedure?
   A. "I will call you after I have gone to the bathroom and urinated."
   B. "I will be sure and flush the toilet after I have voided."
   C. "As soon as I void, the nurse will catheterize me."
   D. "The nurse will leave the catheter in place after the procedure."

2. When obtaining a health history from Katie about her urinary status, the nurse asks the following questions except:
   A. "Are you going to the bathroom frequently?"
   B. "Have you noticed blood in your urine?"
   C. "Do you have a discharge from your vagina after intercourse?"
   D. "What is your fluid intake during the day?"

3. In a renal clearance there are two substances found in the blood that are routinely used to evaluate renal function. The effective indicators of renal function are:
   A. blood urea and GFR.
   B. BUN and serum creatinine.
   C. GFR and BUN.
   D. uric acid levels and creatinine.

4. You are asked to obtain a sterile urine sample from an elderly patient with dementia. The first action should be to:
   A. cleanse the perineal area.
   B. label the container.
   C. place the client in the dorsal recumbent position.
   D. obtain all the supplies needed.

5. A 24-hour urine test is also known as a:
   A. blood urea nitrogen test.
   B. GFR.
   C. creatinine clearance test.
   D. KUB.

6. The physician has ordered a 24-hour urine test for a client with renal disease. The test is to begin at 6 A.M. At what time should the client empty his bladder and discard the urine?
   A. 5 A.M.
   B. 5:30 A.M.
   C. 6 A.M.
   D. The client does not discard any urine.

7. Nursing care for the patient to evaluate urinary retention and incontinence includes all of the following except:
   A. administering pain medications.
   B. using an uroflowmeter.
   C. obtaining a specimen.
   D. measuring urine output.

8. A urinalysis has just been received on the unit for Mr. Kattes. The nurse is aware that a normal urinalysis should not have:
   A. ketones—negative.
   B. protein—3+.
   C. WBC—0-5/HPF.
   D. glucose—negative.

9. Ultrasound examination of the bladder or kidneys is a noninvasive examination that requires:
   A. the client to ingest dye to see the organs.
   B. an empty stomach.
   C. no preparation of the client.
   D. a full bladder.

10. When teaching a client about a renal scan, the nurse informs her that she must increase fluid intake:
    A. before and after the scan.
    B. 4 hours before the scan.
    C. after the scan only.
    D. before the scan only.

# CRITICAL THINKING EXERCISE

Read the following situation. Unscramble the words and define each term. Answer the questions using the nursing process of assessment, diagnosis, planning, implementation, and evaluation.

Intravenous pyelography (IVP) uses a *ttsrncoa dmmuie* and x-rays to evaluate the urinary tract. The contrast medium is injected intravenously. It is *dteelifr* from the blood by the *yksinde,* allowing x-rays to show the contrast entering the kidney pelvis, flowing through the *rreetus,* and into the bladder. This allows evaluation of *nlear* function (by measuring the time required for filtration) and the position, size, shape, and structure of urinary tract organs.

1. What are some other imaging studies used to determine urinary status?
2. Name at least three nursing responsibilities for intravenous pyelography.
3. Document two nursing diagnoses that would be appropriate for a client undergoing imaging studies.

# Chapter 32

# Caring for Clients with Renal and Urinary Tract Disorders

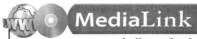

## MediaLink
### www.prenhall.com/burke

Use the address above to access the free, interactive Companion Website created for this textbook. Get hints, instant feedback, and textbook references to chapter-related NCLEX-style questions. Link to other interesting sites.

**Audio Glossary:**

Use the Companion Website, or the CD-ROM disk enclosed with your textbook, to hear the pronunciation of key terms in this chapter.

The renal and urinary systems are vital in the management of waste products that are generated by cell metabolism. This system also plays a major role in the regulation of water and acid-base balance. Client responses depend on the severity of the disorder. Any change in the function of the renal and urinary system has a major impact on daily living.

## ANATOMY AND PHYSIOLOGY

Match each term with its appropriate definition.

| | |
|---|---|
| 1. _____ Incontinence | A. Pelvic floor muscle exercises |
| 2. _____ Retention | B. An inflammatory disorder affecting the renal pelvis |
| 3. _____ Kegel's | C. Involuntary urination |
| 4. _____ Credé method | D. Increased blood levels of nitrogenous wastes, including urea and creatinine |
| 5. _____ Cystitis | E. Disruption to normal urine flow |
| 6. _____ Pyelonephritis | F. The most common cause of obstructed urine flow |
| 7. _____ Glomerulonephritis | G. Applying pressure over the symphysis pubis with the fingers of one or both hands to promote complete bladder emptying |
| 8. _____ Azotemia | H. Damage to glomerular membranes and severe protein loss in the urine |
| 9. _____ Nephrotic syndrome | I. The most common UTI |
| 10. _____ Urolithiasis | J. May be an acute or a chronic disorder |

## FILL IN THE BLANK

Fill in the blanks with the appropriate word or phrase.

1.  A 46-year-old female is concerned that she "wets herself" every time she sneezes. The nurse realizes that this condition could be contributed to a form of incontinence called _____.

2.  A client who has been taking an antidiuretic complains that he dribbles as he is racing to the bathroom. This type of incontinence is known as _____.

3.  A physician has examined an elderly client and informs him that he has an enlarged prostate. The medical term for this condition is called _____.

4.  Your client complains of lower abdominal pain and thick urine. Inspection of his urine sample reveals some blood. The most probable diagnosis for this client might be _____.

5.  A diabetic client arrives in the emergency room complaining that he has not urinated in 24 hours. The urinalysis is positive for high amounts of protein. Based on his medical history, the nurse anticipates the physician may diagnose _____.

6.  A client is seen in the clinic for severe right flank pain and a decreased urine output. Her history is negative for major health problems except hyperparathyroidism. The nurse suspects that this client may be experiencing _____.

7.  Mr. Patrick has just returned from a kidney CT scan. The radiologist's notes indicate an abnormally dilated renal pelvis and calyx in the right kidney. You anticipate that the doctor may diagnose _____.

## MULTIPLE CHOICE

Circle the answer that best completes the following statements.

1.  Which of the following is the most important point to remember when performing a urinary catheterization?
    A.  Assess the amount and color of the initial drainage.
    B.  Provide perineal care before performing the procedure.
    C.  Use sterile technique when inserting the catheter.
    D.  Do not drain more than 800 mL of urine from the bladder.

2.  A middle-aged female client is having a minor problem with stress incontinence. Which of the following nursing interventions would not be included in the nursing care plan?
    A.  Monitor intake and output.
    B.  Teach Kegel exercises.
    C.  Try to hold urine as long as possible before going to the bathroom.
    D.  Limit beverages after the evening meal.

3. The nurse is teaching a young female how to decrease the risk for a UTI. If all of the following are true, which of these statements should have the highest priority?
   A. Do not use bubble bath.
   B. Wipe from front to back.
   C. Wipe from back to front.
   D. Empty the bladder at least every 2 hours.

4. A client asks the nurse about complementary therapies for preventing a UTI. Which of the following fruits would be recommended for this client?
   A. blueberries
   B. grape juice
   C. oranges
   D. pineapple

5. A 28-year-old client has been admitted to the orthopedic floor after sustaining multiple rib fractures in a motorcycle accident. The physician should be notified if the patient develops:
   A. bruising on the chest wall.
   B. a fever of 100 degrees.
   C. oliguria.
   D. an increased appetite.

6. A client receiving Gantrisin for a UTI has developed a rash several hours after taking the first dose. The nurse's best response to this development is:
   A. "The rash is normal. It will go away in a few days."
   B. "You didn't tell me that you were allergic to a sulfa drug!"
   C. "Don't take anymore of the medication. I will notify the doctor."
   D. "I should have looked at your chart before I gave you the mediation."

7. Which of the following should be included in the teaching plan for a patient with an order for Pyridium?
   A. Take the medication for at least 3 days.
   B. Take the drug on an empty stomach.
   C. The medication will clear up the infection in 1 week.
   D. Wear a peripad to protect your underwear.

8. A client has been ordered a low-purine diet. The dietary department calls you to confirm the choices made on the menu. You realize that your client needs further teaching because he ordered:
   A. crab.
   B. tuna.
   C. fried trout.
   D. liver.

9. Which symptom is the client with bladder cancer most likely to exhibit?
   A. painless hematuria
   B. urinary frequency
   C. dysuria
   D. back pain

10. A client has been admitted for major trauma to the pelvis. The physician tells you that she is hypovolemic and orders an IV NS at 150 mL/hour. Based on this information, you should monitor closely for signs of:
    A. acute renal failure.
    B. spontaneous pneumothorax.
    C. chronic renal failure.
    D. urolithiasis.

## CRITICAL THINKING EXERCISE

Read the following situation. Unscramble the words and define each term. Answer the questions using the nursing process of assessment, diagnosis, planning, implementation, and evaluation.

Mr. Forrester, age 68, has presented to the clinic for nausea, apathy, weakness, and fatigue. His history includes a previous myocardial infarction 7 years ago and recent diagnosis of adult-onset insulin-dependent diabetes. A lab workup shows an elevated *NUB* and *umsre rinineteac*. The physician orders a diet to limit *zotmiaae*. *Dimesorefu* is ordered to begin immediately.

1. What medical diagnosis do you anticipate will be documented by the doctor?
2. Discuss the rationale for monitoring the blood pressure every 4 hours.
3. Document two nursing diagnoses that would be appropriate for this client.
4. Why did the physician order this particular diet?

# Chapter 33

# The Reproductive System and Assessment

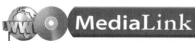

**MediaLink**

www.prenhall.com/burke

Use the address above to access the free, interactive Companion Website created for this textbook. Get hints, instant feedback, and textbook references to chapter-related NCLEX-style questions. Link to other interesting sites.

**Audio Glossary:**

Use the Companion Website, or the CD-ROM disk enclosed with your textbook, to hear the pronunciation of key terms in this chapter.

The major function of the reproductive system is to ensure survival of the species. The primary reproductive organs (gonads) consist of the ovaries and testes. These organs are responsible for the production of egg and sperm cells (gametes) and for the production of hormones. The hormones function in the maturation of the reproductive system and development of sexual characteristics, and they play an important role in regulating the normal physiology of the reproductive system.

## ANATOMY AND PHYSIOLOGY

Match each term with its appropriate definition.

1. __A__ Testes
2. __D__ Scrotum
3. __E__ Spermatogenesis
4. __G__ Epididymis
5. __F__ Testosterone
6. __B__ Ovaries
7. __I__ Estrogen
8. __J__ Progesterone
9. __H__ Fallopian tubes
10. __C__ Uterus

A. Produce sperm and testosterone
B. Produce the female hormones
C. Skin fold over the tip of the penis
D. Pouch that regulates the temperature of the testes
E. Sperm production
F. Male sex hormone
G. Cordlike structure that provides storage of sperm
H. Excretory duct of the testes
I. Steroid hormone essential to the development and maintenance of secondary sex characteristics
J. Hormone that affects breast glandular tissue and the endometrium

# FILL IN THE BLANK

Fill in the blanks with the appropriate word or phrase.

1. An _erection_ occurs when a reflex triggers the parasympathetic nervous system to stimulate arteriolar vasodilation, filling erectile tissue with blood.
2. Estrogens affect serum cholesterol and _HDL_ levels.
3. _Androgens_ (produced in small amounts by the adrenal glands as well as the ovaries) are responsible for normal hair growth patterns at puberty and also have metabolic effects.
4. The _cervix_ is a firm structure that softens in response to hormones during pregnancy.
5. Vaginal mucus is relatively acidic and _bacteriostatic_
6. When assessing a client's reproductive status the nurse knows to first ask about the _presenting problem_ (for both male and female clients).
7. For clients born in the 1940s and 1950s, an important question to ask during your assessment is about possible intrauterine exposure to _diethylstilbesterol_ This drug was used to prevent miscarriage and has been linked to an increased risk for urinary tract deformity and sterility in men, and cervical and vaginal cancer in women.

# MULTIPLE CHOICE

Circle the answer that best completes the following statements.

1. While palpating the inguinal and groin areas of her male patient the nurse knows she is checking for a possible:
   A. STI.
    B. BPH.
   C. hernia.
   D. testicular injury.
2. The nurse knows that when palpating the breast for discharge, the nipples must be
   A. pinched.
   B. rolled.
   C. pulled.
   D. compressed.
3. What is the correct position of a female when assessing the vagina?
   A. supine.
   B. lithotomy.
   C. semi-Fowler's.
   D. knees to chest.

4. Tumors that are too small to be detected by clinical breast exam or self-breast exam can be identified by:
   A. mammography.
   B. x-ray.
   C. CT scan.
   D. MRI.

5. When teaching a client about laparoscopy the nurse must remember to tell the client that the night before the exam she must:
   A. eat.
   B. keep her bladder full.
   C. douche.
   D. discuss the treatment methods with her spouse.

6. Instruct the patient having mammography that 5 to 7 days before the exam she must avoid caffeine and:
   A. carbonated drinks.
   B. blueberries.
   C. purines.
   D. methylzanthines.

7. Colposcopy can identify early premalignant changes in cervical tissue, and is performed when abnormal results are found on:
   A. CT.
   B. endoscopy.
   C. Pap smear.
   D. MRI.

8. In men, the urethra and penis both serve as organs for urine elimination and ejaculation of:
   A. sperm.
   B. bacteria.
   C. oocytes.
   D. enzymes.

9. Bill has been complaining of a loss in libido. His serum testosterone level is 500 ng/dL. Normal serum levels are:
   A. 650–2000 ng/dL.
   B. 280–1100 ng/dL.
   C. 150–500 ng/dL.
   D. 1–50 ng/dL.

10. What could be another possible problem with Bill's loss of libido?
    A. drinking
    B. medications
    C. mental
    D. all of the above

## CRITICAL THINKING EXERCISE

Read the following situation. Unscramble the words and define each term. Answer the questions using the nursing process of assessment, diagnosis, planning, implementation, and evaluation.

Although the *trrseutuc* of the *prctveeourdi* systems in men and women are very different, their *nnuftoisc* are the same: reproduction, sexual *reeslupa*, and development of secondary *lxaesu* characteristics.

1. Spermatogenesis begins with puberty and continues throughout a man's life, with several hundred million sperm produced daily. Explain the process.

2. Discuss the menstrual cycle.

3. Define colposcopy and discuss the procedure.

# Chapter 34

# Caring for Male Clients with Reproductive System Disorders

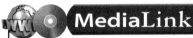

**MediaLink**

**www.prenhall.com/burke**

Use the address above to access the free, interactive Companion Website created for this textbook. Get hints, instant feedback, and textbook references to chapter-related NCLEX-style questions. Link to other interesting sites.

**Audio Glossary:**

Use the Companion Website, or the CD-ROM disk enclosed with your textbook, to hear the pronunciation of key terms in this chapter.

The reproductive system is necessary for procreation. It is responsible for the hormone that produces male sexual characteristics, such as a deep voice and facial hair. Many illnesses and injuries can result in infertility and sterility. Assisting the male patient to cope with these changes is a primary nursing function.

## ANATOMY AND PHYSIOLOGY

Match each term with its appropriate definition.

1. __D__ BPH
2. __G__ Adenocarcinoma
3. __E__ Orchiectomy
4. __C__ Brachytherapy
5. __I__ Prostatitis
6. __J__ Testicular torsion

7. __H__ Cremasteric reflex
8. __B__ Cryptorchidism

9. __F__ Epididymitis

10. __A__ Orchitis

A. Can occur as a complication of mumps
B. Failure of one or both testes to descend through the inguinal ring into the scrotum
C. Implants of radioactive seeds
D. Enlargement of the prostate gland BPH
E. Removal of the testes
F. Usually caused by an infection spread from the bladder, urethra, prostate gland, or seminal vesicles
G. Tumor arising from glandular epithelial cells
H. Retraction of the testicles when the skin on the inside of the thigh is stroked
I. Often associated with lower urinary tract infections
J. Twisting of the testes and spermatic cord

## FILL IN THE BLANK

Fill in the blanks with the appropriate word or phrase.

1. An elderly client presents to the clinic with complaints of nocturia and dribbling. He tells you that he always feels as if his bladder is not empty. This client may be diagnosed with ___BPH___.

2. Mr. Blakely, age 62, reports pain after ejaculation. His vital signs are T-101.2, P-98, R-18, BP-162/78. The physician orders urine and prostate secretion cultures. Mr. Blakely will most likely be diagnosed with _prostatitis_.

3. A 32-year-old African American male has scheduled a routine physical. During the rectal exam, the physician notices that the prostate is hard and enlarged. He orders a PSA test. You suspect that this client may have _prostate cancer_.

4. A young mother is concerned that her child has only one testicle. Based on your knowledge of the male reproductive system, you suspect that the child will be diagnosed with ___cryptorchidism___.

5. A 14-year-old male is brought to the emergency room with severe perineal pain. His father tells you that the client was playing football when the pain began. On inspection, you note that the cremasteric reflex is depressed. You suspect that the young man might be experiencing _testicular torsion_

6. The physician has ordered an ultrasound on a client who presents with an enlarged scrotum. His medical history is insignificant except for epididymitis several weeks ago. The nurse anticipates that the ultrasound will show a _hydrocele_.

7. A 45-year-old client tells his physician that he does not want to have any more children. Instead of using contraceptives, he asks the doctor to perform a _vasectomy_.

## MULTIPLE CHOICE

Circle the answer that best completes the following statements.

1. The nurse has instructed a male client in testicular self-examination. Further teaching is required when the clients says:
   A. "The day I do the exam should be the same day each month."
   B. "I should perform the exam in the shower."
   C. "My testicles should feel soft and walnut-size."
   D. "I will check myself before I have sexual intercourse."

2. You are bathing a male client and notice that he is not circumcised. You pull back the foreskin. After you have cleansed the penis, which of the following must be done?
   A. Have the client empty his bladder.
   B. Separate the foreskin.
   C. Clean the anal area.
   D. Document the bath on the nursing notes.

3. Which of the following clients has an increased risk of developing priapism?
    A. 22-year-old male with spinal cord trauma
    B. 35-year-old male with testicular injury
    C. 62-year-old male with BPH
    D. 84-year-old male with impotence

4. The nursing assistant reports that Mr. Peterson has a sore on his penis. He denies any pain. Your best response should be:
    A. "Okay, just be sure and wash him real good."
    B. "I'll be there in a few minutes to take a look at the sore."
    C. "It's probably nothing. Just document it on the nurse's notes."
    D. "It's probably cancer. I'll let the doctor know right away."

5. A client has been diagnosed with erectile dysfunction. If all of the following are appropriate nursing interventions, which should have the highest priority?
    A. Actively listen to your client's concerns.
    B. Teach the client about the condition.
    C. Explain to the client the importance of pelvic floor exercises.
    D. Discuss the treatment methods.

6. When preparing a client for a transrectal ultrasound-guided biopsy of the prostate, the teaching plan should include which of these instructions?
    A. Client will be fully unconscious during the procedure.
    B. An informed consent is not necessary.
    C. Hematuria and bloody streaks are expected several days after the procedure.
    D. Advise the client to continue on his daily dose of aspirin.

7. Which of these statements, if made by the client diagnosed with prostate cancer, would support a nursing diagnosis of Deficient Knowledge?
    A. "There isn't much hope for me, is there?"
    B. "My doctor said I might have some impotence problems after my surgery."
    C. "The hormone therapy won't cure my cancer."
    D. "If I don't get treated, my cancer might go to my lungs."

8. A client is being treated for prostatitis. The nurse should include which of the following diagnoses in the care plan?
    A. Ineffective Protection related to depressed immune system
    B. Fear related to possible death
    C. Activity Intolerance related to fatigue
    D. Disturbed Body Image related to physical changes

9. The nurse is explaining various approaches to a prostatectomy. She would be correct in stating that a suprapubic prostatectomy is done through:
    A. an incision between the scrotum and anus.
    B. an abdominal incision into the bladder.
    C. an abdominal incision with the bladder remaining intact.
    D. an insertion of a Foley catheter.

10. A client is receiving Viagra. The nurse should plan to observe for side effects, which include:
   A. phimosis.
   B. hypertension.
   C. hypokalemia.
   D. hypotension.

11. Which of these measures should be included in the care plan for a client who is recovering from a TURP?
   A. Use clean technique when handling the drainage system.
   B. Frequently assess catheter patency.
   C. Obtain intake and output every 24 hours.
   D. Maintain the CBI to keep the output cherry red.

12. A client presents with complaints that he has no sexual desire. You anticipate that the physician may order a:
   A. psychologic consult.
   B. testosterone level.
   C. routine urinalysis.
   D. PSA.

13. A client asks you what complementary therapies are available for BPH. Your best response should be:
   A. "I can't talk about other treatments, that's the doctor's job."
   B. "Yoga can help you to relax."
   C. "Saw palmetto grass has been known to reduce the symptoms."
   D. "Flomax helps to relax the smooth muscle."

14. Which nursing intervention would be the most appropriate to meet the expected outcome of "client will wake up less frequently during the night" for a patient who has BPH?
   A. Advise client to restrict alcohol intake.
   B. Provide information about his condition.
   C. Determine his level of anxiety.
   D. Provide pain measures during the day.

15. The patient who is at the highest risk for orchitis is the:
   A. 10-year-old male with measles.
   B. 38-year-old male with HIV.
   C. 42-year-old male with prostate cancer.
   D. 48-year-old male with mumps.

## CRITICAL THINKING EXERCISE

Read the following situation. Unscramble the words and define each term. Answer the questions using the nursing process of assessment, diagnosis, planning, implementation, and evaluation.

A 38-year-old client is suspected of having testicular cancer. His medical history includes a family history of cancer and *simdtorchicryp*. The doctor orders several lab tests, including *palha proteintofe* and *caltic hydroeeedasng*. An *traulnouds* is ordered to rule out other causes of the mass.

1. The diagnosis is confirmed. List three possible medical treatments.
2. Discuss the nursing interventions for the diagnosis Ineffective Sexuality Patterns.
3. What information should be taught to this client after his treatment?
4. What would you include in the documentation if surgery is performed?

# Chapter 35

# Caring for Female Clients with Reproductive System Disorders

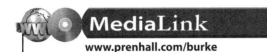

**MediaLink**

**www.prenhall.com/burke**

Use the address above to access the free, interactive Companion Website created for this textbook. Get hints, instant feedback, and textbook references to chapter-related NCLEX-style questions. Link to other interesting sites.

**Audio Glossary:**

Use the Companion Website, or the CD-ROM disk enclosed with your textbook, to hear the pronunciation of key terms in this chapter.

The reproductive system in the female can develop both minor and life-threatening conditions and diseases. The proper functioning of this system is linked to the well-being of the woman. The nurse must respond in an empathetic and sensitive manner when dealing with these changes in the female body.

## ANATOMY AND PHYSIOLOGY

Match each term with its appropriate definition.

1. __B__ Climacteric
2. __D__ Dyspareunia
3. __F__ PMS
4. __A__ Dysmenorrhea
5. __E__ DUB
6. __H__ Hysterectomy
7. __J__ Endometriosis
8. __I__ PCOS
9. __G__ Hirsutism
10. __C__ Fibroids

A. Pain associated with menstruation
B. Period during which menstruation permanently ceases
C. Benign uterine or cervical tumors
D. Pain during sexual intercourse
E. Vaginal bleeding that is abnormal in amount, duration, or time of occurrence
F. A symptom complex of irritability, depression, edema, and breast tenderness preceding menses
G. Excessive hair growth
H. Removal of the uterus
I. An endocrine disorder in which LH, estrogen, and androgen hormone levels are higher than normal, and FSH levels are low
J. Endometrial tissue is found outside the uterus

## FILL IN THE BLANK

Fill in the blanks with the appropriate word or phrase.

1. A young girl is being seen in the clinic for a routine breast exam. The physician notices several small, painless lumps. The client tells him that the lumps go away and then return, especially during her period. The most appropriate diagnosis for this client will be ___fibrocystic Breast A's___.

2. A client, who recently had a baby, complains of sore, swollen, and reddened breasts. It is likely that this client has developed ___mastitis___.

3. A 26-year-old female asks the nurse why she gets so irritable and depressed before her period begins each month. The nurse explains that this condition is referred to as ___PMS___.

4. A client complains of severe cramping during her menses. She also reports a headache and breast tenderness. The most likely diagnosis for this client will be ___primary dysmenorrhea___.

5. Mrs. Sawyer, age 50, tells you that she is having "hot flashes" and has gained 6 pounds during the last month. You recognize that these are symptoms of ___menopause___.

6. A 45-year-old female has been seen in the clinic for urinary frequency, increased bladder infections during the last year, and complaints of difficulty voiding. The physician tells the client that he can see part of her bladder in the vagina. This condition is known as ___cystocele___.

7. Miss Lorie reports to the clinic with complaints of painful intercourse and painful urination. She tells you that she has "terrible" back pain and cramps during her period. The physician feels several firm nodules in her pelvic cavity during his examination. A probable medical diagnosis for this client might be ___Endometriosis___.

## MULTIPLE CHOICE

Circle the answer that best completes the following statements.

1. The nurse is teaching a group of middle school girls the signs of breast cancer. Which of the following would she not include in the lecture?
   A. nipple discharge
   B. unusual lump in the axilla
   C. small, hard, painless lump in the breast
   D. brown area around the nipple

2. A client, who is scheduled for a core-needle biopsy, may need further instruction if she says:
   A. "The doctor will numb my breast."
   B. "I will lie on my back during the procedure."
   C. "Some of my breast tissue will be removed using a needle."
   D. "I can take a mild painkiller when I go home."

3. You are explaining to your patient why she has a swollen abdomen and upper arm pain following a laparoscopy. The best explanation would be:
   A. "Carbon monoxide is blown into the abdominal cavity."
   B. "The pain is coming from the surgical incision site."
   C. "The surgeon had to insert a larger instrument to see inside the abdomen."
   D. "It is caused by carbon dioxide. It allows better visualization of internal organs."

4. A 52-year-old client is upset about the onset of menopause. She asks the nurse how she can cope with the symptoms. The best response should be:
   A. "Avoid drinking alcohol or caffeine."
   B. "Everyone has to go through these changes."
   C. "Splash your face with warm water to relax your muscles."
   D. "Keep the room warm, especially at night."

5. The nurse is assisting the physician in obtaining a cervical smear. She knows that the patient should be placed in this position:
   A. Sim's
   B. lithotomy
   C. supine
   D. side-lying

6. A client presents to the emergency room with a temperature of 103°F and vomiting. Your assessment reveals hypotension and peeling skin on her palms and feet. There is a foul-smelling discharge from her vagina. The client states that she is on her menses and has a tampon in place. Your next action would be to:
   A. place the client in the lithotomy position.
   B. ask the client to remove the tampon.
   C. ask the client if she is pregnant.
   D. remove the tampon.

7. The nurse recognizes that which factor in the client's history is the most important etiological factor in developing cervical cancer?
   A. intercourse using a latex condom
   B. monogamous relationship
   C. infection with HPV
   D. poor hygiene

8. Tamoxifen is most often used for the client with breast cancer because it:
   A. inhibits growth of the tumor by blocking estrogen receptor sites.
   B. replaces lost estrogen needed for cancer protection.
   C. reduces the risk of endometrial cancer.
   D. decreases the spread of breast cancer.

9. A client tells the nurse that she has a fishy-smelling, "milk-like" discharge from her vagina. The nurse suspects that this client has:
   A. atrophic vaginitis.
   B. candidiasis.
   C. trichomoniasis.
   D. simple vaginitis.

10. Which of the following clients is most likely to develop breast cancer in her lifetime?
    A. a client with a familial history of colon cancer
    B. a client who started her menstrual period at 14 years of age
    C. a client who had multiple chest x-rays before she was 30 years old
    D. a client who had her first child at the age of 22

11. Upon admission to the medical floor, the nurse should give highest priority to meeting which need of a client diagnosed with PID?
    A. information related to the prevention of PID
    B. pain control
    C. insertion of a Foley catheter
    D. ordering the daily meals

12. A postmastectomy client refuses to raise her arm above her head because of the presence of a JP drain. The nurse should tell the client:
    A. "You have to exercise your arm to keep it from getting stiff."
    B. "I know it is painful, but the arm needs limbering up."
    C. "You are right. You need to wait until the drains are out to raise your arm."
    D. "Let me get you some pain medication first."

13. In preparing a care plan for a client diagnosed with dysfunctional uterine bleeding, it is most important for the nurse to include a goal that addresses the need for:
    A. sexual function concerns.
    B. increased compliance with the medication regime.
    C. information on how to promote conception.
    D. wound care management.

14. A client has been told that abnormal cells were seen in her initial Pap test. The next action taken by the nurse should be to:
    A. prepare the client for a hysterectomy.
    B. ask the client if she has any questions about the repeat Pap test.
    C. begin an IV of NS in preparation for cauterization of the abnormal cells.
    D. ask the client to sign another consent form.

15. The physician suspects that a client has ovarian cancer. Which of the following lab tests might he order to confirm his diagnosis?
    A. PSA
    B. CA 125
    C. WBC
    D. HGB

## CRITICAL THINKING EXERCISE

Read the following situation. Unscramble the words and define each term. Answer the questions using the nursing process of assessment, diagnosis, planning, implementation, and evaluation.

A 58-year-old client has been diagnosed with *vaseniiv caromanic* of the left breast. Inspection reveals a *Puae d'rangeo* skin texture, *pilenp tractioner,* and a nipple discharge in the left breast. The physician tells the client that the most effective way to manage this cancer is to perform *beastr-vinecronsg* surgery. The client is unsure about the surgery and asks for more options.

1. Which nursing diagnosis best reflects the client's concern?
2. List four nursing interventions that would assist the client in deciding on an option.
3. The client finally agrees to the partial mastectomy. What information should be provided to the client and her family?
4. What information should you document in your nurse's notes relating to your teaching session?

# Chapter 36

# Caring for Clients with Sexually Transmitted Infections

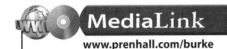

## MediaLink
**www.prenhall.com/burke**

Use the address above to access the free, interactive Companion Website created for this textbook. Get hints, instant feedback, and textbook references to chapter-related NCLEX-style questions. Link to other interesting sites.

**Audio Glossary:**
Use the Companion Website, or the CD-ROM disk enclosed with your textbook, to hear the pronunciation of key terms in this chapter.

Sexually transmitted infections are a diverse group of infections spread through the sexual activity of an infected individual. STIs represent a significant public health problem. The social stigma that surrounds these infections creates many hardships on both the clients and their sexual partners.

## ANATOMY AND PHYSIOLOGY

Match each term with its appropriate definition.

| | | | |
|---|---|---|---|
| 1. _____ Abstinence | A. | Painless ulcer |
| 2. _____ HPV | B. | Slang word for gonorrhea |
| 3. _____ Genital herpes | C. | Venereal Disease Research Laboratory |
| 4. _____ Syphilis | D. | Inflammation of the pelvis |
| 5. _____ Prodromal symptoms | E. | Human papilloma virus |
| 6. _____ Zithromax | F. | Spirochete *Treponema pallidum* |
| 7. _____ Clap | G. | Voluntarily refraining from sexual intercourse |
| 8. _____ Chancre | H. | Herpes simplex 2 virus |
| 9. _____ VDRL | I. | Used to treat chlamydia |
| 10. _____ PID | J. | Warning signals of an impending outbreak |

## FILL IN THE BLANK

Fill in the blanks with the appropriate word or phrase.

1. A male client presents with dysuria, urethral discharge, and testicular pain. He tells you that he had unprotected sex several weeks ago. The nurse suspects that this client has contracted _____.

2. A young client complains of "cuts" in her genital area. She admits to having sex without a condom on several occasions. Inspection reveals several small blisters on the labia. This client may be diagnosed with _____.

3. Your 20-year-old male client has three cauliflower-like growths on the tip of his penis. He complains that he is having difficulty urinating. The most likely diagnosis for this client is _____.

4. A young girl presents to the clinic with severe abdominal pain. Inspection reveals a vaginal discharge. The client tells you that it "hurts" when she goes to the bathroom. This client may have contracted a gram-negative diplococcus known as _____.

5. A client presents with a skin rash on his palms, mucous patches in his mouth, and generalized lymphadenopathy. The physician diagnoses him with secondary _____.

6. A male client has been diagnosed with chlamydia. He is complaining of scrotal pain and swelling. The most likely complication that has developed in this client is _____.

7. A 28-year-old female is being seen in the clinic for a routine Pap test. Her history indicates that she is infected with the herpes virus. Presently, there are no visible lesions. This period of time is called _____.

## MULTIPLE CHOICE

Circle the answer that best completes the following statements.

1. Miss Doyle is examined by the nurse practitioner. The diagnosis is chlamydia. Which of the following interventions would best meet the need of preventing transmission of the organism?
   A. Encourage her partner to get medical attention.
   B. Recommend abstinence while the lesions are healing.
   C. Provide social and emotional support.
   D. Explain the life cycle of chlamydia.

2. A nurse is teaching a sex education class to a group of high school students. To gain a better understanding of their level of knowledge, the nurse asks the students to tell her the name of the most common STI. The correct response should be:
   A. syphilis.
   B. chlamydia.
   C. gonorrhea.
   D. genital herpes.

3. A client admits that he forgets to take his medication prescribed for his gonorrhea. The most effective method to overcome this noncompliance would be to:
   A. call him on the telephone as a reminder.
   B. make an appointment with his case worker.
   C. provide extensive education about his infection.
   D. administer a single dose of medication as ordered.

4. A young man is seen in the emergency room for a profuse and purulent urethral discharge. It is important that the nurse gather information related to:
   A. previous infections.
   B. all sexual contacts.
   C. a history of bladder infections.
   D. recent sexual contacts.

5. After assessing an 18-year-old client, the nurse makes the diagnosis of Health Maintenance, Ineffective. The nurse understands that further teaching is necessary because the client:
   A. has a stable monogamous relationship with her boyfriend.
   B. has never been tested for chlamydia.
   C. has had annual Pap smears.
   D. has multiple sex partners.

6. Mr. Black was diagnosed with gonorrhea and has been treated with a single dose of Rocephin IM. He is given a prescription for doxycycline to take at home. The nurse explains that this combination of antibiotics is prescribed to:
   A. treat any coexisting chlamydial infection.
   B. eliminate resistant strains of gonorrhea.
   C. prevent the development of resistant organisms.
   D. prevent reinfection.

7. Sally Hart has primary syphilis. While caring for her the nurse should:
   A. wear gloves when taking her vital signs.
   B. place the client in isolation.
   C. assess the feet for the presence of blisters.
   D. discuss safer sex practices.

8. The nurse suspects that the client does not understand the disease process of genital herpes when he says:
   A. "As long as I use the medication, I won't infect anyone."
   B. "I have to abstain from having sex when the lesions are present."
   C. "Burow's solution can be used to cleanse the sores."
   D. "I need to purchase some boxer shorts and wear them during the outbreak."

9. A young client tells you that her girlfriend said that "a person would get cancer if they had the papilloma virus." Your best response should be:
   A. "Your girlfriend isn't your doctor."
   B. "There is a greater risk of cervical cancer for those infected with HPV."
   C. "I've never heard of that."
   D. "That idea is just a myth. Just ignore her."

10. A client is being treated for chlamydia. The nurse knows that the teaching has been effective when the client states:
    A. "One injection of penicillin will cure me."
    B. "Use of a spermicidal foam will protect me from further infections."
    C. "Even if I don't get treated, the chlamydia will eventually go away."
    D. "I need to tell my boyfriend so he can get treated."

11. A 24-year-old patient tells you that her boyfriend left her because she has genital warts. She says that he "thought they were disgusting." Based on this information the nurse makes a diagnosis of:
    A. Ineffective Individual Coping.
    B. Anxiety.
    C. Risk for Infection.
    D. Disturbed Body Image.

12. You are collecting data from the chart of a client, age 17, in order to assist in the development of the nursing care plan. You note that this client has been pregnant three times. If all of the following are risk factors for contracting an STI, which should be discussed first?
    A. use of oral contraceptives
    B. adolescent sexual activity
    C. multiple sex partners
    D. unprotected sexual activity

13. The nurse is discussing discharge instructions with a client who has the "clap." The most important point that should be emphasized is:
    A. take all of the prescribed medication.
    B. use a condom for sexual intercourse.
    C. encourage sexual partners to be treated.
    D. return for follow-up appointment.

14. The risk for contracting any STI is directly related to:
    A. number of sexual partners.
    B. lifestyle.
    C. age.
    D. gender.

15. Which of the following must be reported to the public health department?
    A. genital herpes
    B. syphilis
    C. chlamydia
    D. trichomoniasis

## CRITICAL THINKING EXERCISE

Read the following situation. Unscramble the words and define each term. Answer the questions using the nursing process of assessment, diagnosis, planning, implementation, and evaluation.

Eve, 20 years old, has come to your clinic seeking treatment for pain and burning on urination. She also tells you that she can't have *courseinert* because of the pain. She is sexually active but does not use any form of birth control. Physical exam shows a yellowish vaginal discharge and abdominal tenderness. She denies having sex with anyone other than her boyfriend but also confides that they had broken up for a few weeks three months ago. Eve is screened for *madyachil* and *heanroogr*. Her physician admits her to the hospital for IV *tancotefe*.

1. What type of diagnostic test would be performed in the clinic?

2. Name two STIs that should be screened for, in addition to chlamydia and gonorrhea.

3. After discharge from the hospital, how would you evaluate the effectiveness of the nursing teaching plan?

4. Document two nursing diagnoses and two interventions for each.

# Chapter 37

# The Nervous System and Assessment

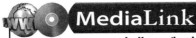

**MediaLink**

**www.prenhall.com/burke**

Use the address above to access the free, interactive Companion Website created for this textbook. Get hints, instant feedback, and textbook references to chapter-related NCLEX-style questions. Link to other interesting sites.

**Audio Glossary:**

Use the Companion Website, or the CD-ROM disk enclosed with your textbook, to hear the pronunciation of key terms in this chapter.

The nervous system is made up of the brain, spinal cord, and their adjacent structures. It is the nervous system that allows the person to interact or react to his or her internal and external environment. Changes that occur in any part of this system frequently are subtle but will have a tremendous impact on the well-being of the client.

## ANATOMY AND PHYSIOLOGY

Match each term with its appropriate definition.

1. _E_ CNS
2. _D_ PNS
3. _B_ Neuron
4. _C_ Axon
5. _G_ Myelin sheath
6. _J_ Synapse
7. _H_ Afferent neurons
8. _I_ Efferent neurons
9. _A_ Dermatome
10. _F_ ANS

A. An area of skin supplied by a single spinal nerve

B. Basic cell of the nervous system

C. Carries impulses away from the cell body

D. The cranial nerves, the spinal nerves, and the autonomic nervous system

E. The brain and spinal cord

F. Responsible for maintaining the body's internal homeostasis

G. A white, fatty substance that protects and insulates axons

H. Carry impulses from the skin and muscles to the CNS

I. Carry impulses from the CNS to the muscles and glands

J. A junction between neurons

## FILL IN THE BLANK

Fill in the blanks with the appropriate word or phrase.

1.  There are two divisions of the autonomic nervous system; the ___SNS___ and the ___PNS___.

2.  The primary function of the eye is to convert patterns of light from the environment into a message that is transmitted via the ___optic nerve___ to the brain.

3.  When the cornea is touched, the eyelids blink and tears are secreted. This is called the ___corneal reflex___.

4.  The ear has two primary functions: ___hearing___ and maintaining ___balance___.

5.  Focused assessment of the client with a possible neurologic disorder begins with identifying the client's ___LOC___.

6.  During Vann's eye exam you notice she has involuntary eye movements. You know from class that this is called ___nystagmus___.

7.  In the older adult the brain atrophies causing slower movement and ___reflexes___ as well as a degree of forgetfulness.

## MULTIPLE CHOICE

Circle the answer that best completes the following statements.

1.  A number of changes in the eye and vision occur with aging. The lens becomes less elastic, affecting near vision. This is known as:
    A.  myopia.
    B.  nystagmus.
    C.  irreversible.
    D.  presbyopia.

2.  Normal cerebrospinal fluid contains:
    A.  a few WBCs.
    B.  a few RBCs.
    C.  +3 protein.
    D.  glucose of 75 mg/dL.

3.  Jeff, the victim of a head injury, has recovered completely except he has trouble speaking. You suspect what area of his brain was affected?
    A.  temporal
    B.  Broca's
    C.  parietal
    D.  Wernicke's

4. Mrs. Mave, 65, had a stroke. She is having difficulty understanding what you say or write to her. You suspect what area of her brain was affected?
   A. Broca's
   B. parietal
   C. Wernicke's
   D. temporal

5. A patient with Bell's palsy most likely has involvement of what cranial nerve?
   A. VII
   B. X
   C. I
   D. XI

6. Loss of fat and subcutaneous tissue around the eyes generally leads to:
   A. difficulty focusing.
   B. reduced light entering the eye.
   C. decreased peripheral vision.
   D. increased risk of infection.

7. Ivan's parents complain of him zoning out for period's of time during the day. Ivan has no recollection of these times and sleeps heavily afterward. You suspect Ivan may have seizures. What test would determine if that diagnosis is correct?
   A. CT
   B. myelography
   C. EMG
   D. MRI

8. This test is used to detect brain cancer, Alzheimer's disease, epilepsy, and Parkinson's disease.
   A. EEG
   B. PET
   C. EMG
   D. CT

9. Tracy, an 18-year-old epileptic, is visibly upset when you go in her room. She is crying and states, "I can't get this gunk out of my hair!" You realize that she has just had a(n):
   A. MRI.
   B. EEG.
   C. PET.
   D. CT.

10. Mark has been complaining about his eye hurting ever since the car accident 2 days ago that broke his windshield. You suspect he may have glass in his eye. What type of test would confirm your suspicions?
    A. visual field test
    B. CT
    C. fluorescein stain
    D. MRI

# CRITICAL THINKING EXERCISE

Read the following situation. Unscramble the words and define each term. Answer the questions using the nursing process of assessment, diagnosis, planning, implementation, and evaluation.

The *nibar* is the control center of the *evuosnr* system. A rigid, bony *klsul* protects the brain from external injury. When the nervous system *sctoialmfnun*, the person may experience acute or chronic *ssddiorer*.

1. Name the three protective meninges of the brain.
2. What are the four regions of the brain?
3. Discuss blood supply to the brain.

# Chapter 38

# Caring for Clients with Intracranial Disorders

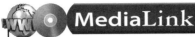

**MediaLink**

www.prenhall.com/burke

Use the address above to access the free, interactive Companion Website created for this textbook. Get hints, instant feedback, and textbook references to chapter-related NCLEX-style questions. Link to other interesting sites.

**Audio Glossary:**

Use the Companion Website, or the CD-ROM disk enclosed with your textbook, to hear the pronunciation of key terms in this chapter.

Intracranial disorders can be acute and life threatening or occur over a long period of time. These disorders often result in long-term problems that affect the client's and family's quality of life.

## ANATOMY AND PHYSIOLOGY

Match each term with its appropriate definition.

1. _H_ TBI
2. _J_ Otorrhea
3. _I_ Battle's sign
4. _B_ ICP
5. _E_ Obtundation
6. _C_ CVA
7. _A_ TIA
8. _G_ Aneurysm
9. _D_ Seizure
10. _F_ Status epilepticus

A. A brief episode of reversible neurologic deficits

B. Pressure exerted within the cranium by the brain, blood, and CSF

C. A brain attack

D. A brief disruption of brain function caused by abnormal electrical activity in the nerve cells of the brain

E. Responds to verbal and tactile stimuli but quickly drifts back to sleep

F. A life-threatening medical emergency that can cause permanent brain damage

G. An abnormal dilation of a cerebral artery

H. A leading cause of death and disability in the United States

I. Bruising over the mastoid process

J. CSF leaks from the ears

# FILL IN THE BLANK

Fill in the blanks with the appropriate word or phrase.

1. Anne is a 12-year-old who is brought to the clinic. Her mother tells you that Anne has had a headache with a stiff neck for 2 days. Today she woke up with vision difficulties and is lethargic. During the exam you note that her neck is flexed. You suspect Anne may have ___meningitis___.

2. A patient with increased intracranial pressure from an infection is receiving Lasix b.i.d., Zantac b.i.d., and Valium prn. An IV of NS 50 cc/hr is infusing in his right arm. The nurse anticipates that the physician will order a medication to decrease the edema, such as ___corticosteroid___.

3. A client with a closed-head injury client is admitted to the hospital for observation. Three hours after his admission, the nurse notes that the nose and ears are oozing a straw-colored fluid. The nurse is aware that this might be ___CSF___.

4. Yesterday a client was admitted with the diagnosis of meningitis. Today he has become increasingly confused and complains of photophobia. His temperature is 103°F. The physician is notified and orders a dose of Valium 10 mg for seizures. The nurse is aware that the client may have developed ___encephalitis___.

5. Andre, age 70, experienced a right-sided CVA 2 days ago. You notice that Andre used his right hand to eat his lunch, but when the phone rang he could not locate it. The phone was on the night stand on the left side of his bed. Based on these observations, you suspect that the client has developed ___neglect syndrome___.

6. An elderly client, diagnosed with a left-sided stroke, is speaking to the nurse but the words are garbled and unclear. This type of speech difficulty is referred to as ___dysarthria___.

7. A 24-year-old male was brought to the emergency room after being involved in a fight with his neighbor. He received several severe blows to his head. The doctor suspects that he has a fractured skull. The client is beginning to lose consciousness. The nurse anticipates that the diagnosis for this client will be ___epidural hematoma___.

# MULTIPLE CHOICE

Circle the answer that best completes the following statements.

1. Why is death a concern when discussing a patient who has developed cerebral edema?
   A. There is decreased fluid to the brain, which causes dehydration.
   B. The force of the excess fluid may cause the brain to herniate.
   C. It is irreversible.
   D. If the edema lasts longer than 24 hours, death is inevitable.

2. You obtain the following results of a client's neurologic assessment: eyes open on command, disjointed conversation ability, unable to answer questions appropriately or to follow instructions. Based on the Glasgow Coma scale this client should be placed at:
   A. 9.
   B. 11.
   C. 15.
   D. 18.

3. Andrew Smythe has been diagnosed with a CVA due to an embolism. He has global aphasia and requires moderate assistance with ADLs. Which of the following would not be an appropriate nursing diagnosis for Mr. Smythe?
   A. Ineffective Tissue Perfusion
   B. Self-Care Deficit
   C. Communication: Verbal, Impaired
   D. Urinary Incontinence, Total

4. Tejas has developed increased intracranial pressure due to an infection. You know to monitor for signs and symptoms of cerebral anoxia because:
   A. infections cause a decrease in blood flow to the brain.
   B. increased ICP creates an increased blood flow to the damaged area.
   C. increased ICP may prevent adequate blood flow to the brain.
   D. cerebral anoxia is a symptom of decreased ICP.

5. Jenny is a 2-year-old child diagnosed with a brain tumor. Which of the following questions would be appropriate to ask the child's mother?
   A. "Has Jenny been having trouble staying awake?"
   B. "Does Jenny have any problems with nausea?"
   C. "Have you noticed any changes in Jenny's speech?"
   D. All of the above questions would be appropriate.

6. Malcolm suffered a head injury after a motorcycle accident. The doctor explains that after a head injury it is not uncommon for a patient to have one or two seizures. If the seizures occur in a chronic pattern, then the patient will likely be diagnosed as having:
   A. Adult-onset seizure disorder.
   B. Convulsion disorder.
   C. Epilepsy.
   D. Seizures.

7. Malcolm has been given a new order for phenytoin 100 mg PO b.i.d. You are providing teaching regarding this medication. What information would you not include?
   A. Driving a vehicle is permitted after the first dose.
   B. CNS or vision changes must be reported to the doctor immediately.
   C. Take the medication with food or after meals.
   D. Blood levels should be checked on a routine basis.

8. Stephanie is a 33-year-old female who developed meningitis after a sinus infection. She has not responded well to the antibiotics and steroids. She asks if she will return to normal after the infection has cleared up. Your best response would be:
   A. "You should recover without complications."
   B. "There is a risk for long-term problems, such as vision or hearing changes."
   C. "Let me call the doctor so he can explain your prognosis to you."
   D. "You will likely be blind and deaf if you recover."

9. Mrs. Deib is 12 hours status postcraniotomy. Which of the following should be included on her nursing care plan?
   A. Keep the head of the bed at 90 degrees.
   B. Encourage Mrs. Deib to eat her prunes every morning.
   C. Obtain vital signs every 8 hours.
   D. Avoid sneezing and straining during bowel movements.

10. Heather is suspected of having a brain tumor. She has become impulsive and has difficulty making decisions. You suspect that her tumor is located in the:
    A. temporal lobe.
    B. frontal lobe.
    C. occipital lobe.
    D. parietal lobe.

11. During the assessment of a patient experiencing headaches, the patient tells the nurse that she has had headaches off and on during the past several years. She also says that she becomes severely nauseated when the pain of the headache begins. Her only management for these headaches has been sleep. The nurse suspects she has:
    A. migraine headaches.
    B. tension headaches.
    C. cluster headaches.
    D. general headaches.

12. The first priority when a client begins to have a grand mal seizure should be to:
    A. time the length of the seizure.
    B. administer Valium to stop the seizure.
    C. place a tongue depressor in the mouth.
    D. maintain an open airway without restricting the client's movements.

13. Altered level of consciousness is likely to be observed in a patient with:
    A. increased ICP.
    B. strokes, head injury, or meningitis.
    C. any injury that causes a decrease of oxygen or glucose to the brain.
    D. injuries that primarily affect the cranial nerves.

14. Which of the following interventions would be appropriate for any intracranial disorder?
    A. bowel management, diuretics, anticoagulants
    B. fall prevention, ADL assistance, bowel management
    C. anticoagulants, fall prevention, ADL assistance
    D. reorientation, caregiver training, fall prevention

15. A client has lost his ability to chew because of a stroke. The nurse knows that the nerve of mastication is called the:

    A. vagus.
    B. abducens.
    C. trigeminal.
    D. trochlear.

## CRITICAL THINKING EXERCISE

Read the following situation. Unscramble the words and define each term. Answer the questions using the nursing process of assessment, diagnosis, planning, implementation, and evaluation.

> Mrs. Wallace, 74 years old, was admitted to the emergency room after falling down several steps at her home. Her diagnoses include a fractured right femur, dehydration, and mild renal insufficiency. The chart also notes a history of CHF, hypertension, and insulin-dependent diabetes. On the fourth day postop, she refuses to get out of bed to participate in physical therapy exercises. When you enter the room, Mrs. Wallace begins to speak in gibberish and her face begins to droop on the left side. Your assessment finds *ssievprexe siaaaph* with *thiarrasid* and left-sided *pleigiameh*. The physician is notified and the final diagnosis is a cerebral vascular accident. He orders a new medication, *toksenaistrep*.

1. Discuss the risk factors that may have contributed to the CVA.
2. List four nursing interventions that you would initiate to prevent aspiration.
3. What was the rationale for the streptokinase order?
4. What information should be documented when assessing a client with a CVA?

# Chapter 39

## Caring for Clients with Degenerative Neurologic and Spinal Cord Disorders

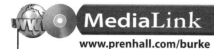

**MediaLink**

**www.prenhall.com/burke**

Use the address above to access the free, interactive Companion Website created for this textbook. Get hints, instant feedback, and textbook references to chapter-related NCLEX-style questions. Link to other interesting sites.

**Audio Glossary:**

Use the Companion Website, or the CD-ROM disk enclosed with your textbook, to hear the pronunciation of key terms in this chapter.

Degenerative neurologic disorders disrupt the central nervous system (CNS) and the peripheral nerves. They can cause devastating physical and emotional changes. The client and family often face lifestyle and role changes and may even experience financial difficulties. The exact cause of these disorders is uncertain. Some may have a genetic or autoimmune cause. The nurse is expected to assist the patient in all aspects of care to help them reach their maximum potential with the limitations that are presented.

## NEUROLOGIC DISORDERS TERMINOLOGY

Match each term with its appropriate definition.

1. __D__ Rhizotomy
2. __J__ Dopamine
3. __E__ Bradykinesia
4. __I__ Sundowning
5. __H__ Chorea
6. __G__ Thymectomy
7. __A__ Fasciculations
8. __B__ Demyelination
9. __F__ Sciatica
10. __C__ Myelography

A. Involuntary contraction of skeletal muscles
B. Destruction or loss of myelin sheath
C. Visualization of spinal cord using x-rays
D. Surgical severing of a nerve root
E. Slowed speech or movement
F. Pain that follows the sciatic nerve
G. Surgical removal of the thymus gland
H. Uncontrollable, jerky movements
I. Increased confusion in evening or late hours
J. Neurotransmitter that inhibits voluntary motor function

# FILL IN THE BLANK

Fill in the blanks with the appropriate word or phrase.

1. A 40-year-old construction worker has been treated for a herniated disk for 6 months. His medical management has included bed rest, physical therapy, and anti-inflammatories. The client is not improving, despite the conservative care. The doctor will probably consider _Spinal fusion_.

2. A patient arrives in your clinic with complaints of arm and leg weakness. She tells you that "it happened so fast." Her medical history reveals that she received the flu vaccine several days ago. After assessing her respiratory status, you suspect that this patient has developed _Guillan Barre Syndrome_.

3. An elderly client tells the office nurse that she can't wash her face or even brush her teeth because of the pain on the right side of her face. She states that she has not been hurt except for a slightly unpleasant trip to the dentist 1 week ago. Based on this information, the nurse believes that this client has _Trigeminal Neuralgia_.

4. A patient arrives in the emergency room after receiving severe injuries from falling off of her horse. She cannot move her legs. The nurse observes urine stains on her clothing. The physician is concerned that there is spinal cord injury at the level of _S1-S5_.

5. Elizabeth has a pronounced droop to her left eyelid and left side of her mouth. She admits to some pain but states that the drooling is more bothersome. She has no weakness in her extremities. Her history reveals the contraction of herpes simplex. Elizabeth most likely will be diagnosed with _Bells Palsy_.

6. A child had been bitten by a raccoon that had wandered into his backyard. The doctor writes an order for an immune globulin (RIg). The nurse realizes that the child is at risk for contracting _Rabies_.

7. A patient enters the clinic. The nurse notices that he appears to have a stiff neck and that a dirty bandage is on his upper arm. The patient tells you that he fell off of a bicycle several weeks ago and that the cut has not healed. The nurse asks about the patient's vaccination history because she suspects _tetanus_.

# MULTIPLE CHOICE

Circle the answer that best completes the following statements.

1. Rodney is recovering from a fracture of the T3–T5 vertebra after a fall. He has made significant progress in rehabilitation and is due to be discharged home. The primary nursing diagnosis for his discharge planning will be:
   A. Risk for Autonomic Dysreflexia.
   B. Risk for Impaired Skin Integrity.
   C. Ineffective Individual Coping.
   D. Self-Care Deficit: Toileting.

2. The primary nursing intervention for a patient with a newly placed Halo vest is:
   A. cleansing the pin sites every 4 hours.
   B. inspecting the pins and traction bars for tightness.
   C. turning the patient every 2 hours.
   D. providing pain relief as needed.

3. Angus is 24 hours status postspinal fusion of L1–L2. Which of the following should be documented on the nursing care plan?
   A. Remove collar during the dressing change.
   B. Ensure the corset is applied correctly.
   C. Assess the donor site at the iliac crest.
   D. Assess the patient for LOC, headache, and blurred vision.

4. You are preparing a patient for a myelography. The patient needs further teaching if he states:
   A. "After the test, I should drink lots of fluids."
   B. "The dye is going to make me feel a bit cool."
   C. "I won't drink anything for several hours before the test."
   D. "I will definitely try to void as soon as I feel the urge."

5. A patient diagnosed with multiple sclerosis is being prepared for discharge. The nurse is assessing the patient's home care. The most important question to ask the patient is:
   A. "Do you understand the disease process for MS?"
   B. "Will you be able to prepare a well-balanced meal?"
   C. "Do you have enough financial resources to help you through this crisis?"
   D. "Is there anyone at home who has a cold?"

6. A 32-year-old woman presents to the emergency room and is diagnosed by the doctor with a cholinergic crisis. Which of the following represents the most appropriate question in order to gain information about this condition?
   A. "Do you feel short of breath?"
   B. "How much of the neostigmine did you take this week?"
   C. "Have you had any nausea or vomiting?"
   D. "Have you experienced any fast heartbeats?"

7. A mother asks the nurse if her child really needs to receive a tetanus vaccine or if there is some other preventive measure that would be more effective. The best response should be:
   A. "He needs the vaccine."
   B. "The vaccine will decrease his chances of developing tetanus."
   C. "If you clean all of his cuts right away, there really is no need for the injection."
   D. "You won't have to worry anymore about tetanus if he gets the shot."

8. Mr. Jones has been taking Haldol for the treatment of a mild psychosis. He displays a shuffling gait, mild hand tremors, and slurred speech. The nurse knows that these symptoms may be clinical manifestations of:
   A. Parkinson's disease.
   B. parkinsonism.
   C. Tourette's syndrome.
   D. Creutzfeldt–Jakob disease.

9. The <u>primary nursing intervention</u> during the assessment of a person with a spinal cord injury is to:
   A. ensure that the person's head remains immobile.
   B. assess the respiratory status.
   C. maintain the airway.
   D. assess for autonomic dysreflexia.

10. Douglas was in a car accident several weeks ago and has now been admitted to the rehabilitation facility for further evaluation of his T3 injury. During his teaching session, the nurse should remind Douglas to:
   A. call the nurse for any severe headache.
   B. report a rise in his blood pressure.
   C. report the sensation of a full bladder.
   D. ask for help when ambulating to the bathroom.

11. Wanda has had a laminectomy 2 hours ago and is complaining of a headache. You logroll her to inspect the dressing on her back. There is a large amount of clear drainage noted on the gauze. Your next action should be to:
   A. remove the dressing to check the incision site.
   B. raise the head of the bed to relieve the headache.
   C. test the drainage with a glucose reagent strip.
   D. call the doctor.

12. An elderly patient, admitted for a hernia repair, has become confused and agitated during the evening shift. The nurse suspects that the patient is suffering from sundowning. Which of the following actions is appropriate for this patient?
   A. Restrain the patient's hands.
   B. Close the door so he won't disturb the other patients.
   C. Document the behavior.
   D. Ask a nursing assistant to stay in the room until a plan of care is formulated.

13. The most effective drug for the treatment of Parkinson's disease is:
   A. Sinemet.
   B. Parlodel.
   C. Permax.
   D. levodopa.

14. A client with <u>severe muscle spasms</u> from a spinal cord injury calls the nurse for any medication that will <u>decrease</u> the pain. The nurse checks the doctor's orders and administers:
   A. diazepam.
   B. Tensilon.
   C. Artane.
   D. Cogentin.

15. Sarah has a complete spinal cord injury at the level of T1. She develops spinal shock. Which of the following are manifestations of this condition?
   A. tachycardia
   B. hypertension
   C. diaphoresis
   D. flaccid paralysis

## CRITICAL THINKING EXERCISE

Read the following situation. Unscramble the words and define each term. Answer the questions using the nursing process of assessment, diagnosis, planning, implementation, and evaluation.

A 58-year-old female has been tentatively diagnosed with *meri'shalez* disease, Stage 1. The doctor has ordered *tarpice* for treatment. In addition, he has ordered several diagnostic tests, which include an *trogramhaloceleeepnc* and a *ticenagm nancereso magingi scna* of the brain. The client's husband is concerned about his wife's memory loss and occasional angry outbursts.

1. Discuss the manifestations of the early stages of Alzheimer's.
2. List two communication techniques that you could teach the client's husband.
3. What self-care deficit interventions would be appropriate for this client?
4. What assessment data should be documented in the client's record?

# Chapter 40

# Caring for Clients with Eye and Ear Disorders

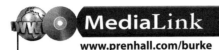

**MediaLink**

www.prenhall.com/burke

Use the address above to access the free, interactive Companion Website created for this textbook. Get hints, instant feedback, and textbook references to chapter-related NCLEX-style questions. Link to other interesting sites.

**Audio Glossary:**
Use the Companion Website, or the CD-ROM disk enclosed with your textbook, to hear the pronunciation of key terms in this chapter.

Vision and hearing are special senses that allow us to experience the world in which we live. The special senses warn us of danger, protect us from injury, and help maintain position sense and balance. Deficits in the special senses may limit self-care, mobility, independence, communication, and relationships with others. Understanding the changes that occur with the aging process will assist the nurse in providing effective care to all age groups.

## ANATOMY AND PHYSIOLOGY

Match each term with its appropriate definition.

1. __A__ Conjunctiva
2. __H__ Depth perception
3. __I__ Iris
4. __E__ Tympanic membrane
5. __B__ Hearing
6. __J__ Pinna
7. __F__ Cerumen
8. __D__ Lacrimal gland
9. __C__ Macula
10. __G__ Pupil

A. Membrane that lines the anterior surface of the eye
B. Perception and interpretation of sound
C. Area of central vision in the retina
D. Produces tears to moisten and irrigate the eye
E. Vibrates and transmits sound to the middle ear
F. Earwax
G. Controls the amount of light that enters the eye
H. Ability to identify distances between objects
I. Colored portion of the eye
J. External portion of the ear

## FILL IN THE BLANK

Fill in the blanks with the appropriate word or phrase.

1.  An elderly man is complaining of the inability to read the newspaper print and tells you that he has difficulty focusing. This client most likely will be diagnosed with _presbyopia_.

2.  John, a 50-year-old with a history of diabetes mellitus and a two- to three-pack-a-day cigarette habit, tells the physician that he is having trouble driving at night because of the glare from oncoming traffic. The physician points out the cloudy lenses to the student nurse. The physician suspects that John is developing _cataracts_.

3.  A client tells the nurse that she has poor peripheral vision, sees blurry rings around lights, and cannot see when the lights are completely cut off. She denies any pain. The nurse believes that this client may have _glaucoma_.

4.  A 3-year-old child has a history of chronic upper respiratory infections. She presents to the clinic with severe pain in her left ear. The physician orders an antibiotic and tells the mother that the child has _otitis media_.

5.  A 72-year-old client complains that he is slowly losing his hearing in the right ear. When you respond to his comment he bends his ear toward the sound of your voice. You recognize that this client is suffering from _presbycusis_.

6.  Gerri is a young girl with a history of chronic middle ear infections. After the fourth visit of the year, the physician tells Gerri's father that he needs to drain the ear in a procedure known as a _myringotomy_.

7.  A client reports that he is always getting "attacks of dizziness." He explains that it is like riding on a merry-go-round, including the nausea feeling. He further adds that his left ear constantly rings. This client is probably suffering from _Meniere's disease_.

## MULTIPLE CHOICE

Circle the answer that best completes the following statements.

1.  The nurse is preparing a discharge instruction sheet for a patient who had ear surgery 2 days ago. Which of the following must be included in this plan?
    A.  Take antiemetics t.i.d.
    B.  Change the inner dressing daily.
    C.  Keep the mouth open when sneezing or coughing.
    D.  Do not bathe until released by the doctor.

2.  A patient with newly diagnosed glaucoma is receiving eyedrops for the first time. After instilling the drops you gently squeeze the bridge of his nose for 1 minute. He asks you why you are pinching his nose. The best response should be:

A. "If I pinch the nose, you won't move around as much."
B. "It keeps more of the medication in your eye."
C. "Pinching the nose increases the blood supply to the eyes."
D. "I'm sorry. I shouldn't have pinched your nose for such a long time."

3. You are responding to an accident in the hospital kitchen. A coworker is bleeding from her right eye. Upon examination you see a small shard of metal penetrating her eye through the eyelid. Your next action is to:
   A. irrigate the eye with normal saline.
   B. remove the object, then irrigate the eye.
   C. place a cup over the injured eye and tell her to keep the other eye closed.
   D. take her to the emergency room.

4. A cataract is:
   A. a clouding of the eye lens.
   B. the filling of the space between the lens and cornea with aqueous humor.
   C. an occluded canal of Schlemm.
   D. incurable and leads to blindness.

5. After eye surgery, a patient is frequently instructed not to bend over for a couple of days because:
   A. eye pressure increases when bending at the waist.
   B. the medication will flow out of the eye.
   C. it may cause the stitches to loosen.
   D. the bending movement will increase the pain.

6. A patient with glaucoma asks how long he must use eyedrops. The nurse responds:
   A. "Sorry, for the rest of your life."
   B. "When the canal of Schlemm opens completely and remains open."
   C. "It all depends on the success of your surgery."
   D. "There is no way to correct your problem, so you must use the drops for life."

7. Xia Zihuen is a young woman with a diagnosis of retinal detachment. You are giving preoperative instructions regarding the corrective surgery. You should first:
   A. provide information about the mydriatic eyedrops.
   B. discuss the types of corrective lens available.
   C. explain that perfect vision may not be possible after the procedure.
   D. assess her language skills and educational level.

8. A young child is more likely to suffer from otitis media than an adult because:
   A. children are more susceptible to inner ear infections.
   B. the eustachian tube is more horizontal in children.
   C. children are more likely to get colds and flus.
   D. it is a common childhood illness.

9. The primary nursing diagnosis for a patient experiencing an acute attack of vertigo is:
   A. Anxiety.
   B. Risk for Aspiration.
   C. Risk for Injury.
   D. Powerlessness.

10. You are teaching a client the proper positioning of the head for instilling eardrops in his right ear. The correct procedure would be to:
    A. lie on the affected side.
    B. tilt the head backward.
    C. tilt the head toward the unaffected side.
    D. tilt the head forward.

11. Which of the following is least likely to develop sensorineural hearing loss?
    A. patient with Meniere's disease
    B. patient with a perforated eardrum
    C. construction worker
    D. patient on high doses of antibiotics

12. The nurse instructs a patient who is using Betoptic eyedrops to check her pulse 1 hour after instillation of the medication. The rationale for this is:
    A. tachycardia is a severe side effect.
    B. the medication is a beta-blocker.
    C. Betoptic is contraindicated in COPD and heart failure patients.
    D. the doctor wants a report on the adverse reactions experienced by the patient.

13. The nurse is conducting a Weber test on a 24-year-old client. He knows that the test is negative if the client hears:
    A. sound in both ears equally.
    B. sound in the right ear only.
    C. sound in the left ear only.
    D. no sound.

14. Which of the following is most likely to develop external otitis media?
    A. Olympic swimmer
    B. football player
    C. karate teacher
    D. hairdresser

15. The nurse is demonstrating the assessment of the six cardinal fields of vision in a continuing education class. A student asks, "What is the purpose of this test?" The nurse should state that the purpose is to:
    A. determine if the patient has vision in those areas of the eye.
    B. determine if the patient is able to follow directions.
    C. assess the smoothness of the eye movement.
    D. assess the function of the extraocular muscles.

## CRITICAL THINKING EXERCISE

Read the following situation. Unscramble the words and define each term. Answer the questions using the nursing process of assessment, diagnosis, planning, implementation, and evaluation.

A 72-year-old client, Mrs. Jasper, is being seen in the clinic for a routine eye examination. You notice that when she is reading, she holds the magazine at arm's length and squints. During the examination, she tells the doctor that her eyes feel so dry and scratchy and that her eyelashes are irritating her left

eye. The doctor makes these notes and diagnoses in the chart: *byopiaresp,*
*opionrent,* early stages of *comagalu, juncvitisitcon.*

1. What type of treatment might be prescribed for the glaucoma?
2. Name two nursing interventions that will decrease the spread of the eye infection.
3. What is included in the assessment of this patient?
4. Why would this patient have a diagnosis of conjunctivitis?

# Chapter 41

# The Musculoskeletal System and Assessment

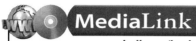

**MediaLink**

www.prenhall.com/burke

Use the address above to access the free, interactive Companion Website created for this textbook. Get hints, instant feedback, and textbook references to chapter-related NCLEX-style questions. Link to other interesting sites.

**Audio Glossary:**

Use the Companion Website, or the CD-ROM disk enclosed with your textbook, to hear the pronunciation of key terms in this chapter.

The musculoskeletal system includes bones and joints of the skeleton, connective tissues such as tendons and ligaments, and the skeletal muscles. The musculoskeletal system allows us to remain upright and to move and protect our vital organs. It is the nurse's responsibility to identify age-related changes and provide objective assessment data related to the musculoskeletal system and its function.

## ANATOMY AND PHYSIOLOGY

Match each term with its appropriate definition.

1. __F__ Osteocytes
2. __E__ Tendons
3. __J__ Skeletal muscle
4. __I__ Yellow bone marrow
5. __B__ Bursae
6. __H__ Osteoblasts
7. __A__ Red bone marrow
8. __D__ Smooth muscle
9. __G__ Ligaments
10. __C__ Osteoclasts

A. Manufactures blood cells and hemoglobin
B. Cushions and protects bony areas
C. Cells that are associated with resorption of bone
D. Provides involuntary movement
E. Connects muscles to bone
F. Cells responsible for bone maintenance
G. Connects bones to bones
H. Cells associated with bone production
I. Contains fat and connective tissue
J. Allows voluntary movement

## FILL IN THE BLANK

Fill in the blanks with the appropriate word or phrase.

1. Bones are covered with __periosteum__, a double-layered connective tissue that contains blood vessels and nerves.

2. Bone remodeling is regulated by _hormones_, the effects of gravity, and mechanical stress from the pull of muscles.

3. Sandra, age 32 and an avid tennis player, comes to the clinic complaining of her right shoulder "clicking and popping" at times when she wakes up in the morning. She denies pain, swelling, or loss of movement, stating, "It's just nerve-wracking!" You suspect there may be decreased _synovial fluid_ in her shoulder.

4. The muscles of the bladder wall, gastrointestinal system, and bronchi are smooth muscle. Their movement is controlled by _internal mechanisms_.

5. Two days ago, Brandon, 42, participated in a 10-mile walk for diabetes. Prior to the walk Brandon, an accountant, received no training or exercise on his own. Today he is complaining of severe thigh and calf pain. You know that Brandon is suffering from a buildup of _lactic acid_ and muscle fatigue related to prolonged strenuous physical activity.

6. Older adults, women in particular, tend to lose bone mass, along with joint and disk cartilage (it dehydrates and loses its flexibility) with aging. Together, these changes contribute to a loss of _height_ and a stooped posture.

7. Posture changes the older adult's center of gravity, increasing the risk for _falls_.

## MULTIPLE CHOICE

Circle the answer that best completes the following statements.

1. When caring for a patient with a leg cast, which of these assessments requires immediate nursing intervention?
   A. cool distal appendages
   B. edematous foot
   C. increased capillary refill
   D. pain on a scale of 6

2. A patient has sustained several rib fractures from falling off of a roof. If all of these interventions are possible, which should have the highest priority?
   A. Administer analgesics as ordered.
   B. Encourage use of incentive spirometer.
   C. Splint chest for breathing or coughing.
   D. Assess respiratory status every 4 hours.

3. A nurse teaches a patient how to care for a sprained ankle. Which of these statements indicates that further teaching is necessary?
   A. "I will keep my leg elevated as much as possible."
   B. "My prescription for my pain medication has been sent to the pharmacy."
   C. "I'm going to use a heating pad this evening."
   D. "My ace bandage is comfortable now."

4. You are assisting the nurse educator in teaching a class on proper range-of-motion techniques. She asks you to demonstrate the movement of pronation. You should:
   A. move in a circle.
   B. turn your palms down.
   C. bend your ankle upward.
   D. turn your foot outward.

5. Which of these nursing interventions is the most important when caring for a patient with a fractured tibia?
   A. neurovascular assessment
   B. administering pain medications
   C. respiratory assessment
   D. cast care

6. Mrs. Dawson states that she is unable to complete normal daily activities because of the pain from her fibromyalgia. The most appropriate response by the nurse is:
   A. "I can ask the doctor to refer you to a psychiatrist for help."
   B. "Do you think the pain is real?"
   C. "I understand that this is painful. Exercise can be helpful."
   D. "You can't continue to depend on drugs to help you."

7. Which of the following behaviors observed by the nurse requires intervention to decrease the risk of back injury?
   A. The patient care technician bends his knees to retrieve the client's slippers.
   B. The nursing assistant is pulling a large equipment cart down the hallway.
   C. A coworker uses a ladder to replace supplies on a top shelf.
   D. A nurse raises the bed to waist height to turn a patient.

8. The nurse is instructing a client and his wife about a bone scan procedure scheduled for the afternoon. Which of the following should be discussed during this session?
   A. NPO status 8 hours before the procedure.
   B. Client will have to drink 8 ounces of contrast medium.
   C. The scan will take at least 30 to 60 minutes to complete.
   D. Radioactive precautions must be taken after the procedure.

9. Maintaining an active lifestyle and specific exercises such as weight training help counteract aging changes, maintain muscle mass, and prevent:
   A. rheumatoid arthritis.
   B. osteoporosis.
   C. fractures.
   D. myeloma.

10. Ken complains of "water on the knee." What two assessments can you do to determine if he actually has extra fluid in his knee joint?
    A. bulge sign and ballottment
    B. Thomas test and bulge sign
    C. ballottment and Thomas test
    D. arthrocentesis and bulge sign

# CRITICAL THINKING EXERCISE

Read the following situation. Unscramble the words and define each term. Answer the questions using the nursing process of assessment, diagnosis, planning, implementation, and evaluation.

*Nvlsyoia* joints are found at all limb articulations. The surfaces of synovial joints are covered by *graacitle,* and the joint cavity is enclosed by a tough, *sborifu* capsule. This *yvtaci* is lined with synovial membrane and filled with synovial *udlif.*

1.  Name the three types of joints and their function.
2.  Discuss the connection between ligaments and tendons.
3.  Discuss the three types of muscle and their function.

# Chapter 42

# Caring for Clients with Musculoskeletal Trauma

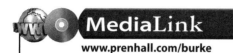

**MediaLink**

**www.prenhall.com/burke**

Use the address above to access the free, interactive Companion Website created for this textbook. Get hints, instant feedback, and textbook references to chapter-related NCLEX-style questions. Link to other interesting sites.

**Audio Glossary:**

Use the Companion Website, or the CD-ROM disk enclosed with your textbook, to hear the pronunciation of key terms in this chapter.

Musculoskeletal trauma ranges from mild to severe. The severity of trauma depends on both the amount of force and the location of impact, because different parts of the body can withstand different amounts of force. Nurses play a major role in trauma prevention by educating the community about safety and injury prevention.

## ANATOMY AND PHYSIOLOGY

Match each term with its appropriate definition.

1. __J__ Trauma

2. __C__ Contusion

3. __G__ Sprain

4. __I__ Strain

5. __A__ Fracture

6. __H__ Compartment syndrome

7. __F__ Reduction

8. __B__ Cast

9. __E__ Traction

10. __D__ Gangrene

A. Occurs when bone is subjected to more force than it can absorb

B. A rigid device used to immobilize broken bones and promote healing

C. Bleeding into soft tissue resulting from blunt force

D. Tissue death that can lead to amputation

E. Uses a straightening or pulling force to return or maintain the fractured bones in normal position

F. Restoration of normal alignment

G. A ligament injury

H. Excess pressure restricts blood vessels and nerves

I. A microscopic tear in the muscle that causes bleeding into the tissues

J. Occurs when tissues are subjected to more force than they are able to absorb

# FILL IN THE BLANK

Fill in the blanks with the appropriate word or phrase.

1. Janice sustained a fracture of the left femur in a skiing accident. She complains of chest pain and SOB. Petechiae appear on her chest. The nurse recognizes Janice may be developing _fat emboli_.

2. A client is complaining of unrelenting pain underneath his arm cast. His fingers are edematous and pale. His capillary refill is greater than 7 seconds. These signs and symptoms may indicate _compartment syndrome_.

3. Your patient begins to complain of leg pain 3 days after she has undergone a repair of her right hip due to a fall. There is definite swelling and redness in the right leg calf. The patient may be developing _DVT_.

4. Mr. Scott, age 86, was found 12 hours after he had fallen from a ladder. When he arrives at the emergency room, the physician tells you that Mr. Scott has a dislocated shoulder and is at risk for developing _femoral head necrosis_.

5. An administrative assistant is seen in the clinic for numbness, tingling, and weakness in the hands. She is unable to hold her pencil without pain. The nurse recognizes that this client may have _CTS_.

6. Kevin's left arm is amputated below the elbow in an industrial accident. Four days following the accident, he insists that his left hand is burning. Kevin is experiencing _phantom pain_.

7. A client who had a below-the-knee amputation 8 months ago is admitted to the hospital for revision of severe flexion of the same knee. Due to the lack of range-of-motion activities, this client has developed _contractures_.

# MULTIPLE CHOICE

Circle the answer that best completes the following statements.

1. A patient is admitted to the hospital with a fractured hip. Which of these statements describes the main goal of therapy?
   A. alleviating pain
   B. maintaining circulation
   C. preventing additional trauma
   D. increasing mobility

2. The nurse is discussing discharge instructions with a patient who has undergone a below-the-knee amputation. Which action by the patient would indicate acceptance of the body part loss?
   A. verbalizing understanding of the dressing change
   B. touching the incision
   C. asking questions related to pain medication
   D. looking at the amputation site

3. A plaster of Paris cast was applied to your patient's left arm several hours ago. You were asked to teach the patient how to care for the cast. Which of the following statements would indicate that the patient <u>understood</u> your instructions?
    A. "Could I borrow a hair dryer to speed the drying process?"
    B. "Wow, my arm is warm."
    C. "Guess I won't need a sling now that I have this cast."
    D. "Look at the indentations in this cast!"

4. The nurse is admitting a patient in the emergency room who sustained an injury while playing soccer. Which of the following clinical manifestations might indicate that the patient's shoulder is dislocated?
    A. edema of the upper arm
    B. pain radiating to the wrist
    C. increased length of the affected arm
    D. bruising in the scapula region

5. Jerry twists his right ankle, injuring several <u>ligaments</u>. This injury is classified as a:
    A. sprain.
    B. strain. (muscles)
    C. contusion.
    D. fracture.

6. A client's wrist is edematous and painful as a result of a sports accident. Initial treatment should include:
    A. elevation and heat application.
    B. elevation and ice application.
    C. elevation and ace bandage only.
    D. elevation and a splint.

7. A fracture that involves protrusion of the bone through the skin is a(n):
    A. complete fracture.
    B. compound fracture.
    C. greenstick fracture.
    D. oblique fracture.

8. A patient has skeletal traction to her left leg. Appropriate nursing action to assist in transporting the patient to the x-ray department would be:
    A. maintain traction during transport.
    B. remove weights before transporting.
    C. place weights on the bed.
    D. secure the weights on the traction frame.

9. Mrs. Carson has had a right hip arthroplasty. A priority nursing intervention during the postoperative phase is to:
    A. maintain the hip in adduction.
    B. maintain the hip in <u>abduction</u>.
    C. maintain the Buck's traction.
    D. perform active ROM on the right leg.

10. A client has an above-the-knee amputation resulting from uncontrolled diabetes. The nurse should recognize that the purpose of using an elastic wrap on the stump is to:
    A. prevent pain.
    B. prevent hemorrhage.
    C. prevent edema.
    D. prevent infection.

## CRITICAL THINKING EXERCISE

Read the following situation. Unscramble the words and define each term. Answer the questions using the nursing process of assessment, diagnosis, planning, implementation, and evaluation.

Tracy was transported to the emergency department of a local hospital following an automobile accident. She sustained a *poundcom carfuret* of the right femur. Her vital signs are stable with the exception of a pulse rate of 110. A temporary cast is applied in the operating room until an *OFIR* can be performed. The physician orders include *cuvasneuroarl* checks every 2 hours, elevation of the extremity, IV antibiotics, and call the physician if any signs of a *atf mesmilob* develop.

1. Discuss the assessment that the physician has specifically ordered.
2. List three nursing diagnoses and prioritize each.
3. List the signs and symptoms of a fat embolism.
4. Document your assessment after Tracy has returned from the recovery room.

# Chapter 43

# Caring for Clients with Musculoskeletal Disorders

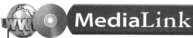
**www.prenhall.com/burke**

Use the address above to access the free, interactive Companion Website created for this textbook. Get hints, instant feedback, and textbook references to chapter-related NCLEX-style questions. Link to other interesting sites.

**Audio Glossary:**

Use the Companion Website, or the CD-ROM disk enclosed with your textbook, to hear the pronunciation of key terms in this chapter.

Musculoskeletal disorders affect clients by causing pain, deformity, and impaired mobility. These manifestations may be mild or severe, chronic or acute. The nurse uses the nursing process to assist the client in coping with the effects of these disorders.

## MUSCULOSKELETAL DISORDERS

Match each term with its appropriate definition.

1. __E__ Ankylosing spondylitis    A. Loss of bone mass
2. __F__ Gout    B. Softening of the bones
3. __G__ Kyphosis    C. Bunion
4. __H__ Rheumatoid arthritis    D. Joint replacement
5. __D__ Arthroplasty    E. Chronic inflammation and stiffening of the spine
6. __I__ Scoliosis    F. Accumulation of uric acid crystals in the joints
7. __B__ Osteomalacia    G. Increased thoracic curvature
8. __C__ Hallux valgus    H. Systemic connective tissue inflammatory disorder
9. __A__ Osteoporosis    I. Lateral curvature of the spine
10. __J__ Arthralgia    J. Joint pain

## FILL IN THE BLANK

Fill in the blanks with the appropriate word or phrase.

1. The school nurse examines a 12-year-old girl. She notes that the student's left shoulder is lower than the right. The nurse suspects that she may have _scoliosis_ _lateral curvature_

2. Mrs. Dennis presents with the following signs and symptoms: anorexia, malaise, joint pain, and a red rash over her nose. The physician will most likely diagnose Mrs. Dennis with _systemic lupus eryth-_

3. A client complains of redness, edema, and severe pain in his right great toe, especially during times of stress. The physician orders a uric acid test. You suspect that this client may be suffering from _Gout_.

4. Mrs. Singer, age 55, is 5'5" tall and weighs 245 pounds. She complains of severe pain and a "grating" sensation in her left knee when she walks. She also reports a sedentary lifestyle. Mrs. Singer is at risk for a type of joint disorder called _Osteoarthritis DJD_

5. An elderly female tells you that she has shrunk during the last few years. She has developed a curvature of her thoracic spine. This client most likely has developed _Osteoporosis_.

6. A 7-year-old child fell from his tree house and sustained an open fracture of his left radius. The site was cleansed and the fracture was reduced in the operating room. Two days following the surgery, the nurse notes that the child's temperature is 103°F and that there is purulent drainage at the incision site. The nurse suspects that the client is at risk for _Osteomyelitis. (bone infection)_

7. A client with severe, chronic rheumatoid arthritis is not responding to his current treatment plan. The doctor debates whether or not to remove the client's circulating antibodies by a therapy known as _plasmapher_. ?

## MULTIPLE CHOICE

Circle the answer that best completes the following statements.

1. Mrs. Montez, age 58, is diagnosed with osteoporosis. The teaching plan should include which of the following points?
   A. Increase weight-bearing exercises.
   B. Increase isometric exercises.
   C. Reduce calcium intake.
   D. Increase protein intake.

2. The nurse informs a client with osteoporosis that a new drug has been prescribed to inhibit bone resorption. Which of the following medications has this action?
   A. sodium fluoride
   B. calcium carbonate
   C. estrogen
   D. alendronate

A D C A
C C D D
B D A B

3. Hanna is diagnosed with SLE. The nurse would be most alarmed if Hanna developed:
   A. painful joints.
   B. severe headaches.
   C. abnormal breath sounds.
   D. weight loss.

4. Hydroxychloroquine has been prescribed for a patient with systemic lupus. Patient teaching should include:
   A. have eye examinations every 6 months.
   B. avoid the use of NSAIDS.
   C. measure output every 8 hours.
   D. document daily weights.

5. A client is prescribed a low-purine diet. The nurse recognizes the need for further teaching if he chooses this food for lunch:
   A. chicken.
   B. milk.
   C. liver.
   D. corn.

6. Your patient has been given a prescription for allopurinol. He calls the clinic to report that a rash has developed on his chest and arms. The nurse's best response should be:
   A. "Don't worry, it will go away in a few days."
   B. "Please stop taking the medication."
   C. "Discontinue the drug and make an appointment with your doctor right away."
   D. "Finish taking the pills and then schedule a follow-up appointment."

7. You are teaching a client about a high-calcium diet. The client understands the instructions if he tells you that the best source of calcium would be:
   A. a seafood platter.
   B. broccoli casserole.
   C. tofu.
   D. whole milk.

8. The nurse is developing a care plan for a patient with gout. The diagnosis is acute pain. Which of the following interventions should be included in the plan of care?
   A. Increase outdoor activity.
   B. Wrap foot with an ace bandage.
   C. Keep the foot warm by covering with a sheet.
   D. Administer analgesics as ordered.

9. Joan went on a vacation in the mountains. One month after her return, she developed malaise, fever, muscle pain, and an unusual skin lesion. You suspect that the doctor will treat Joan for:
   A. Rocky mountain spotted fever.
   B. Lyme disease.
   C. rabies.
   D. malaria.

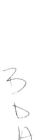

10. A client is diagnosed with the most common malignant bone tissue tumor of the long bones. Based on your knowledge of bone tumors, you suspect that the tumor will be classified as:

    A. multiple myeloma.
    B. Ewing's sarcoma.
    C. chondrosarcoma.
    D. osteosarcoma.

11. The nurse is reviewing a client's medical records and notes that the ESR is elevated and the rheumatoid factor is positive. Using this knowledge, the nurse believes that the doctor will make a diagnosis of:

    A. rheumatoid arthritis.
    B. ankylosing spondylitis.
    C. muscular dystrophy.
    D. Paget's disease.

12. Gold salt therapy is prescribed for a client with rheumatoid arthritis. The primary function of this medication is to:

    A. reduce pain.
    B. reduce joint deformities.
    C. reduce inflammation.
    D. reduce infection.

## CRITICAL THINKING EXERCISE

Read the following situation. Unscramble the words and define each term. Answer the questions using the nursing process of assessment, diagnosis, planning, implementation, and evaluation.

Mary Jones, age 68, is diagnosed with *teoathrrtisios* in both knees. She complains of severe pain when bending, walking, or attempting to sit down in a chair. Physical exam reveals enlargement of both knees. She describes *pretcusi* on movement. The physician has indicated that Mary will have to have bilateral knee *plastirotesath*. He has ordered *phencetaanomi* for pain.

1. List four nursing interventions that you would recommend for Mary to help with her mobility problems.

2. Explain the use of acetaminophen in her treatment.

3. Begin to teach Mary about her surgery. List three preoperative teaching points.

4. What documentation is necessary after Mary has returned from surgery?

# Chapter 44

# The Integumentary System and Assessment

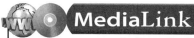

The skin provides an external covering for the body, separating the body's organs and tissues from the external environment. The skin contains receptors for touch and sensation, helps regulate body temperature, and assists in fluid and electrolyte balance. Nurses focus on how to assess and educate clients in skin care.

## INTEGUMENTARY DISORDERS

Match each term with its appropriate definition.

1. _____ Melanin
2. _____ Epidermis
3. _____ Keratin
4. _____ Dermis

5. _____ Erythema

6. _____ Vitiligo
7. _____ Edema

8. _____ Clubbing

9. _____ Lentigines

10. _____ Macule

A. Flat, nonpalpable change in skin color
B. Reddening of the skin
C. Angle of nail base is greater than 180 degrees
D. Outermost part of the skin made of epithelial cells
E. Protect nerve endings in the dermis from the damaging effects of ultraviolet light
F. Hyperpigmentation called "liver spots"
G. An abnormal, patchy loss of melanin, over the face, hands, and groin
H. A fibrous, water-repellent protein that makes the epidermis tough and protective
I. Deeper layer of skin made up of a flexible connective tissue
J. Accumulation of fluid in the body's tissues

## FILL IN THE BLANK

Fill in the blanks with the appropriate word or phrase.

1. The skin and its appendages of glands, nails, and hair make up the system known as the _____.

2. The layer of skin that is supplied with nerve fibers and lymphatic vessels is called the _____.

3. The yellow-orange pigment that combines with melanin to produce the golden hues in people of Asian descent is known as _____.

4. Secretion of the ecrine glands, which contain water, antibodies, sodium, and other elements, is referred to as_____.

5. Ceruminous glands, located in the external ear, secrete a sticky substance which is called _____.

6. Another name for dry skin is _____.

7. Skin color may be influenced by emotions or illness. A change in skin color that may result when an individual is embarrassed or running a fever is called _____.

## MULTIPLE CHOICE

Circle the answer that best completes the following statements.

1. Caucasians have a pinkish skin tone because of:
   A. profuse erythema.
   B. blood leakage.
   C. red blood cells underneath skin.
   D. melanin.

2. The nurse is reviewing a client's record and notes that the medical history includes psoriasis. Based on her knowledge of this condition, the nurse does not expect to find which of the following clinical manifestations?
   A. discoloration and pitting of the nailbeds
   B. silvery, white scaly patches on the scalp, elbows, knees, and sacral area
   C. gray areas of plaque
   D. diffuse red rash

3. During inspection of a client's skin, the nurse observes an irregularly shaped, heavily pigmented "mole." The nurse's next action should be to:
   A. ask the patient if he was aware of the mole.
   B. document the size, color, and appearance in the chart.
   C. notify the physician immediately.
   D. check the medical history in the records.

4. A teenager asks his nurse what is causing his acne. The nurse most appropriately responds by saying:
   A. "It's caused by eating lots of fried foods and chocolate."
   B. "It is caused by clogged oil glands."
   C. "The exact cause is not known."
   D. "It is caused by excessive sunlight and heat."

5. To soothe the itching of acne lesions, the nurse might suggest which of the following interventions?
   A. Cleanse lesions with soap and hot water.
   B. Teach the client to rub instead of scratching the lesions.
   C. Apply a soothing, sweet-smelling lotion to the face.
   D. Rub the face briskly with a towel after cleansing.

6. A client is admitted to the neuro floor after experiencing a CVA with resulting left-sided paralysis. The most important nursing intervention at this time should be to:
   A. turn every 2 hours.
   B. place in a low-Fowler's position.
   C. limit fluid intake.
   D. consult with physical therapist to begin gait training.

7. Randy, 45, has been diagnosed with cirrhosis of the liver. He has a yellow pigment to his skin. You know this is called:
   A. jaundice.
   B. melaninic.
   C. keratotic.
   D. cyanotic.

8. You notice that your patient's oxygen is not connected. His lips are starting to turn blue and he is lethargic. As you hook his oxygen back up and call the respiratory therapist, you realize his lips are:
   A. jaundiced.
   B. melanin.
   C. keratin.
   D. cyanotic.

9. You notice your neighbor, 57, outside in her garden. When you go outside to talk to her, she seems confused; thinking she may be dehydrated you check her skin for:
   A. bruising.
   B. rashes.
   C. erythema.
   D. tenting.

10. Red splinter hemorrhages and pigmented bands on nails are normal in 90% of:
    A. Caucasians.
    B. African Americans.
    C. Hispanics.
    D. Chinese.

# CRITICAL THINKING EXERCISE

Read the following situation. Unscramble the words and define each term. Answer the questions using the nursing process of assessment, diagnosis, planning, implementation, and evaluation.

A variety of normal *ksin* changes are seen in the older adult. Loss of subcutaneous *utssei,* dermal thinning, and decreased *ttleasiicy* may cause wrinkles and sagging of the skin. The skin is thinner, and *rrugto* is decreased. Older adults are unable to respond to heat or cold quickly, increasing their risk for heat stroke and *ytehhpeoiamr*.

1. List three other age-related changes in older adults.
2. Discuss melanocyte production in older adults.
3. Discuss hair and nail growth in aging.

# Chapter 45

# Caring for Clients with Skin Disorders

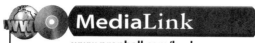

**MediaLink**

www.prenhall.com/burke

Use the address above to access the free, interactive Companion Website created for this textbook. Get hints, instant feedback, and textbook references to chapter-related NCLEX-style questions. Link to other interesting sites.

**Audio Glossary:**

Use the Companion Website, or the CD-ROM disk enclosed with your textbook, to hear the pronunciation of key terms in this chapter.

Disorders of the skin may be minor, such as itching and burning, or they may be so severe that infection and disfigurement lead to major complications. Clients with cancer of the skin may be faced with metastatic disease, which could be fatal. The nurse should be prepared to assist the client in coping with these skin changes.

## COMMON SKIN DISORDERS

Match each term with its appropriate definition.

| | | | |
|---|---|---|---|
| 1. _____ Pruritus | | A. | Fever blister or cold sore |
| 2. _____ Cellulitis | | B. | Caused by the human papilloma virus |
| 3. _____ Herpes zoster | | C. | Infection at skin surface extending into hair follicle |
| 4. _____ Acne | | D. | Shingles |
| 5. _____ Verrucae | | E. | Athlete's foot |
| 6. _____ Pediculosis | | F. | Subjective itching sensation |
| 7. _____ Exfoliative dermatitis | | G. | Skin disorder of the sebaceous glands |
| 8. _____ Herpes simplex | | H. | Infestation with lice |
| 9. _____ Tinea pedis | | I. | Characterized by peeling skin |
| 10. _____ Folliculitis | | J. | Diffuse inflammation of the skin layers |

## FILL IN THE BLANK

Fill in the blanks with the appropriate word or phrase.

1.   _____ that persists may interrupt sleep patterns, because the itching sensation is often more intense at night.

2. _____ is a chronic, noninfectious skin disorder. It is characterized by raised, reddened, round circumscribed plaques of varied size,
   covered by silvery white scales.

3. _____ dermatitis is caused by a hypersensitivity response or
   chemical irritation.

4. _____ dermatitis is an inflammatory skin disorder characterized
   by excessive peeling or shedding of skin.

5. A disorder of the sebaceous glands is called _____.

6. Acne _____ is common in adolescents and young to middle-aged adults.

7. Teach clients using oral corticosteroids to never stop taking the medication
   _____.

## MULTIPLE CHOICE

Circle the answer that best completes the following statements.

1. Mr. Williams is admitted to the hospital for treatment of acute cellulitis
   caused by a spider bite. He asks the nurse to explain what the term means.
   The nurse plans to base a response on the understanding that cellulitis is a(n):
   A. skin infection that extends into the subcutaneous fat.
   B. acute superficial infection.
   C. inflammation of the epidermis.
   D. epidermal infection caused by staphylococcus.

2. The nurse is assessing a patient and notices eczema on the back of his neck
   and bilateral knees. Based on her knowledge of this condition, the nurse
   expects to find:
   A. gray areas of plaque.
   B. diffuse red rash.
   C. discoloration and pitting edema.
   D. silvery, white scaly patches.

3. The physician has just diagnosed a client with herpes simplex Type I. The
   nurse expects the medication ordered will be:
   A. triple antibiotic.
   B. Bactroban.
   C. acyclovir.
   D. actinex.

4. Retin-A is prescribed for the treatment of acne. The nurse questions the
   order if the medication is ordered for a:
   A. 12-year-old diagnosed with asthma.
   B. 15-year-old male diagnosed with cystic fibrosis.
   C. 20-year-old diagnosed with eczema.
   D. 25-year-old male diagnosed with HIV.

5. Marvin states he will not go the prom because of his acute acne. The most appropriate response by the nurse would be:
   A. "Lots of kids your age have zits. That's no reason to stay at home."
   B. "Can't you get a date?"
   C. "I can tell this upsets you. Please tell me more."
   D. "The lesions will be cleared by prom time next year."

6. Ms. Taylor has contracted genital herpes. Which of the following has the highest priority when teaching the client about the disease?
   A. Take the medication as ordered.
   B. Avoid oral sex.
   C. Wash hands before eating a meal.
   D. The disease is incurable.

7. A breast cancer patient develops shingles following chemotherapy treatment. A priority nursing diagnosis for this patient would be:
   A. Therapeutic Regimen Management, Ineffective.
   B. Disturbed Body Image
   C. Deficient Knowledge
   D. Self-Care Deficit

8. Discharge instructions for a patient diagnosed with cellulitis should include:
   A. apply cool compresses t.i.d.
   B. discontinue the medication when the symptoms disappear.
   C. cover draining lesions with a sterile dressing.
   D. keep skin moist at all times.

9. Mr. Yale is diagnosed with basal cell carcinoma of the left cheek. Which of the following indicates a need for further teaching?
   A. "I need to wear a hat when I go outside in the sun."
   B. "I need to get my affairs in order, since I don't have much time left."
   C. "The cancer can return after treatment."
   D. "The treatment is usually effective."

10. A neighbor calls you during the evening and asks you to look at her child's head. When you asked about the problem, the neighbor says that "rice grains" are stuck to the roots of the hair. From your knowledge of lice, you would anticipate that the physician will diagnose:
    A. scabies.
    B. pediculosis corporis.
    C. pediculosis capitis.
    D. tinea pedis.

## CRITICAL THINKING EXERCISE

Read the following situation. Unscramble the words and define each term. Answer the questions using the nursing process of assessment, diagnosis, planning, implementation, and evaluation.

A 24-year-old male has been semicomatose for 10 days following a motor vehicle crash. The physical assessment reveals the following data: T-101, P-110, R-16, BP-142/80; skin is moist with patches of *psoiariss* on the elbows.

You note that he scratches his genitals frequently. The physician has diagnosed this client with *peserh leximps II* and *dylmataonoc minatauca*. You are also concerned about the potential for the development of *ssurepre cerslu*. The charge nurse has established a nursing diagnosis of Risk for Impaired Skin Integrity. A goal, prevention of skin breakdown, is established.

1. List five nursing interventions to help this patient meet the goal.

2. What precautions should the nursing staff implement when caring for this client?

3. Name two medications that you anticipate will be ordered by the doctor.

4. Document the skin assessment in narrative form.

# Chapter 46

## Caring for Clients with Burns

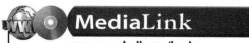

www.prenhall.com/burke

Use the address above to access the free, interactive Companion Website created for this textbook. Get hints, instant feedback, and textbook references to chapter-related NCLEX-style questions. Link to other interesting sites.

**Audio Glossary:**

Use the Companion Website, or the CD-ROM disk enclosed with your textbook, to hear the pronunciation of key terms in this chapter.

Caring for clients with burn injuries involves critical nursing observation and treatment skills. The client may be at risk for multiple complications involving fluid loss, infection, and multisystem failure. Scarring that results from burn injuries requires the nurse to intervene in the psychologic as well as the physical needs of the client.

## BURN INJURY TERMINOLOGY

Match each term with its appropriate definition.

1. _____ Eschar
2. _____ Superficial partial-thickness burn
3. _____ Radiation burn
4. _____ Full-thickness burn
5. _____ Chemical burn
6. _____ Electrical burn
7. _____ Superficial
8. _____ Deep partial-thickness burn
9. _____ Debridement
10. _____ Thermal burn

A. Results from acidic or basic agents
B. Entire dermis plus hair follicles
C. Removal of dead tissue from wound
D. Caused by brief exposure or contact
E. Exposure to dry heat
F. Hard crust that forms over wound
G. Sunburn
H. Severity depends on duration of voltage
I. Extends to subcutaneous fat, muscle, bone
J. Involves only epidermis

## FILL IN THE BLANK

Fill in the blanks with the appropriate word or phrase.

1. Immediately following a burn, massive fluid shifts occur in the extravascular spaces. The resulting decreased intravascular fluid volume is called

   _____.

2. Clients with burns are at increased risk for infection. The state of impaired cell-mediated and humoral-mediated systems is referred to as _____.

3. Inhalation injuries produce a decreased arterial oxyhemoglobin and a state of tissue hypoxia. Oxygen is displaced by a colorless gas known as _____.

4. A severely burned client complains of abdominal pain and nausea. His stools are bloody. This client may be suffering from _____.

5. Massive fluid loss following a severe burn injury results in dehydration and oliguria. The nurse is aware that the client should maintain a urinary output of _____.

6. Continuous assessment of a client's blood oxygen saturation level may be accomplished using an instrument known as a _____.

7. A method for determining the extent of surface area damage on a burn victim is referred to as the _____.

## MULTIPLE CHOICE

Circle the answer that best completes the following statements.

1. A client sustains second- and third-degree burns over 45% of his body. The nursing care immediately following this burn injury is:
   A. prevention of infection.
   B. fluid resuscitation.
   C. preservation of body image.
   D. maintenance of urinary output.

2. The nurse describes the client's burn injury in the medical record as "pale, waxy and moist, with large blister formation." The client states that the pain is at level 5. The depth of injury is most likely:
   A. full thickness.
   B. superficial.
   C. superficial partial thickness.
   D. deep partial thickness.

3. The emergent stage of burn injury treatment includes:
   A. closure of the burn wound.
   B. wound debridement.
   C. estimating the extent of the burn.
   D. skin grafting.

4. Mr. Andrews, age 68, is receiving fluid resuscitation of Ringer's lactate at 250 mL/hr. Which of the following indicates a complication of fluid therapy?
   A. urinary output of 85 mL/hour
   B. complaints of abdominal pain
   C. crackles in lung bases
   D. edema in the burn areas

5. A major complication of a severe burn is infection. If all of the following nursing interventions are placed on the care plan, which would be the highest priority?
   A. Monitor and record body temperature every 2 hours.
   B. Review WBC counts.
   C. Maintain a high-calorie diet.
   D. Use aseptic technique.

6. A 7-year-old child sustains a thermal burn to her face when she trips over an open gas heater. Your first action should be to:
   A. determine the depth of the burn.
   B. assess the respiratory status.
   C. provide pain medication.
   D. read the doctor's orders.

7. Your client is receiving Ensure at 60 mL/hr via a nasogastric tube. Which of the following interventions should be written on the nursing care plan?
   A. Record daily weights.
   B. Replace feeding tube every 24 hours.
   C. Administer a stool softener once a day.
   D. Increase the rate when the client complains of hunger.

8. Mrs. Jones has sustained burns over 55% of her body. She complains of nausea and has been throwing up a dark, green fluid. Your next action would be to:
   A. assess bowel sounds.
   B. insert a nasogastric tube.
   C. administer an antiemetic.
   D. notify the charge nurse.

9. The nurse is reviewing the lab work for a client with severe burns over 60% of his body. The HGB is 10.8 and the HCT is 55%. The nurse recognizes that these lab values may indicate:
   A. blood loss.
   B. nutritional deficit.
   C. hemolysis and fluid shifts.
   D. infection.

10. A client is complaining of severe pain after receiving second- and third-degree burns to her chest and lower extremities. The nurse expects to administer medication by the:
    A. intravenous route.
    B. intramuscular route.
    C. subcutaneous route.
    D. oral route.

11. Silver nitrate wet dressings are used as a topical treatment for a client with a full-thickness burn to the left arm. Client teaching should include:
    A. the dressing will be painful.
    B. the dressing will be removed every 2 hours.
    C. the dressing will feel warm.
    D. the dressing will cause the skin to turn black.

12. The primary goal of the rehabilitative stage should be to:
    A. prevent contractures.
    B. prevent infection.
    C. manage the pain.
    D. increase the nutritional status.

13. You have been assigned to assist the physician in the debridement of a burn wound located on a client's forehead. Which of the following actions would not be appropriate for this client?
    A. Administer pain medications 30 minutes before the procedure.
    B. Wash the wound with Hibiclens.
    C. Provide a pair of surgical scissors to remove eschar.
    D. Trim any hair that might interfere with the procedure.

14. Mr. Kaiser will be going to surgery for a heterograft. He asks the nurse, "Where does the doctor get the graft material?" The nurse should state:
    A. "We have the local university tissue bank send a piece from a cadaver."
    B. "The surgeon will take a piece of skin from your thigh."
    C. "Your daughter has already volunteered to provide a graft."
    D. "The graft is usually taken from a pig skin."

15. A client with 60% burn injuries will be receiving a nutritional diet. You expect that the physician will initially order:
    A. a 2500-calorie, high-protein, high-carbohydrate, low-fat diet.
    B. TPN.
    C. enteral feedings through a small-bore tube.
    D. gastrostomy feedings.

## CRITICAL THINKING EXERCISE

Read the following situation. Unscramble the words and define each term. Answer the questions using the nursing process of assessment, diagnosis, planning, implementation, and evaluation.

Mr. Sanchez has received burns to his face, neck, chest, left back, and both upper extremities. The burns to the hands and face are deep partial-thickness burns. The remaining are full-thickness burns. His treatments include fluid resuscitation, *orerthapyhyd, bridetnemde,* and the topical application of *dineselav.* The physician anticipates the need to perform an *tomyesorahc.* Nursing orders are to place Mr. Sanchez on $O_2$ 5 L per nasal cannula, insert a Foley catheter, and begin IV fluids via the triple lumen central line.

1. Using the "rule of nines," determine the percentage of Mr. Sanchez's burns.

2. List three potential complications that you should anticipate.

3. Develop a plan of care.

4. After you have completed the orders provided by the physician, what should your nursing documentation contain?

# Chapter 47

# Mental Health and Assessment

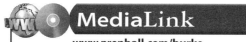

**www.prenhall.com/burke**

Use the address above to access the free, interactive Companion Website created for this textbook. Get hints, instant feedback, and textbook references to chapter-related NCLEX-style questions. Link to other interesting sites.

**Audio Glossary:**

Use the Companion Website, or the CD-ROM disk enclosed with your textbook, to hear the pronunciation of key terms in this chapter.

One out of every 5 American adults suffers from a diagnosable mental disorder in any given year. This represents more than 44 million people. Nurses diagnose and treat problems affecting all aspects of the client: body, mind, and spirit. Because mental health is an important aspect of the health of each person, assessment of the mental health status of clients is an essential part of nursing practice.

## MENTAL HEALTH TERMINOLOGY

Match each term with its appropriate definition.

| | | | |
|---|---|---|---|
| 1. _____ Insight | | A. | Chemical messengers that conduct impulses from one neuron to the next |
| 2. _____ Concrete thinking | | B. | Attitudes, beliefs, customs, and behaviors passed from one generation to the next |
| 3. _____ Neurotransmitter | | C. | Nerve cell |
| 4. _____ Neuron | | D. | Self-understanding |
| 5. _____ Synapse | | E. | Rapidly changing emotional expressions |
| 6. _____ Stigma | | F. | Literally or without creativity |
| 7. _____ Psychosocial | | G. | Negative attitude marking people with certain conditions as less valuable |
| 8. _____ Culture | | H. | Space between the axon and its target cell's dendrite |
| 9. _____ Self-concept | | I. | Refers to things that affect psychologic and social functioning |
| 10. _____ Labile | | J. | How we relate to ourselves and to others |

## FILL IN THE BLANK

Fill in the blanks with the appropriate word or phrase.

1. Elaine, 44, keeps repeating everything you say in your initial assessment. You realize this is known as _____.

2. A decrease in _____ affects sleep and thought processes.

3. You ask your client, "What might work better for you?" As a nurse you realize this form of questioning tells you how your client plans to _____.

4. The question, "Has the surgery changed the way you feel about yourself?" deals with _____.

5. Self-concept may be assessed by asking _____ or _____.

6. At least _____ of the elderly in nursing homes suffer from a mental disorder.

7. _____ is the most common mental disorder.

## MULTIPLE CHOICE

Circle the answer that best completes the following statements.

1. Nancy is a 22-year-old patient diagnosed with depression. When assessing the patient's past coping behaviors the nurse knows to ask:
   A. "Why are you depressed?"
   B. "When the stress gets really bad, what do you do?"
   C. "So, what happened this time?"
   D. "Don't you realize how blessed you are?"

2. A neurotransmitter thought to be decreased in depression is:
   A. GABA.
   B. norepinephrine.
   C. acetylcholine.
   D. FTGA.

3. To assess short-term memory, ask the client to remember three words when you begin the mental status assessment. If the client remembers accurately, short-term memory is said to be intact when you ask what the three words were:
   A. 10 seconds later.
   B. 30 minutes later.
   C. 5–10 minutes later.
   D. 5 hours later.

4. One way to assess abstract thinking ability is to ask the client to interpret a proverb. This simple assessment can shed light on the client's:
   A. thought process.
   B. emotional state.
   C. life experiences.
   D. behavior.

5. An inflated appraisal of one's abilities, power, or knowledge is termed:
   A. labile.
   B. neologism.
   C. euphoria.
   D. grandiosity.

6. A young woman comes into the clinic with chronic pancreatitis. She smiles when you tell a joke, but her overall affect is sad. Because nurses treat clients holistically, an important aspect of nursing in this case is to also promote:
   A. no pain.
   B. patient advocacy.
   C. physical strength.
   D. mental health.

7. Mental disorders are diagnosed according to the diagnostic criteria published in:
   A. *Taber's*.
   B. the DHHS.
   C. the DSM-IV-TR.
   D. the PDR.

8. The leading cause of disability in developed countries by 2020 is projected to be:
   A. psychosis.
   B. major depression.
   C. schizophrenia.
   D. anxiety.

9. As client advocates, nurses should stop using the negative labels about people who have mental illnesses, and:
   A. educate the public.
   B. have a staff meeting.
   C. preach to the choir.
   D. educate each other.

10. A more specific assessment that is appropriate for a client with mental disorders is called a:
    A. psychosocial assessment.
    B. complete assessment.
    C. mental status examination.
    D. focused examination.

## CRITICAL THINKING EXERCISE

Read the following situation. Unscramble the words and define each term. Answer the questions using the nursing process of assessment, diagnosis, planning, implementation, and evaluation.

Psychosocial is a broad term that refers to things that affect *ysclhoogicp* and social *niitnucfngo*. When a client is admitted to a health care facility, the nurse may do an *iiintla* psychosocial *mtssaessen* in addition to the physical assessment. Each *ciitlyfa* will have its own format.

1. Name the aspects of psychologic functioning and of social functioning.
2. Information about a client's family and culture are important parts of the psychosocial assessment. Why?
3. What is culture and how does it influence behavior?

# Chapter 48

# Caring for Clients with Psychotic Disorders

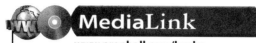

Psychosis is a major feature of schizophrenia, which is the most common thought disorder. Affected people experience psychosis; disorganization of the personality; and an impaired ability to interpret reality, to relate to self and others, and to function in daily life. Nursing practice is concerned with the client's response to illness, so the client's signs and symptoms are of interest to nurses.

## THOUGHT DISORDERS

Match each term with its appropriate definition.

1. _____ Psychosis
2. _____ Schizophrenia
3. _____ Familial

4. _____ Hallucination
5. _____ Delusion
6. _____ Alogia
7. _____ Avolition

8. _____ Prodromal
9. _____ Milieu
10. _____ Opisthotonos

A. Sensory perceptions that seem very real but occur without external stimuli
B. A complex disorder of the brain
C. A thought disorder that causes delusions, hallucinations, disorganized speech, or disorganized behavior
D. Early symptoms
E. Fixed false beliefs
F. Decreased amount and richness of speech
G. Generalized muscle spasms that result in arching of the back and neck
H. Therapeutic environment
I. A lack of motivation
J. A disease that occurs in families

## FILL IN THE BLANK

Fill in the blanks with the appropriate word or phrase.

1.  _____ affects approximately 1% of the adult population.

2.  Four types of _____ function are affected by schizophrenia: attention, executive function, insight, and short-term memory.

3.  Mr. Filch has been scheduled for an EEG. You suspect he may be schizophrenic based on your interview with him. If you are correct his EEG results will show abnormal _____.

4.  More than 100 studies in 34 countries have shown a 5% to 8% increase in the birth rate of people with schizophrenia during the months of _____.

5.  The pathophysiology most pertinent to nursing care involves the excess of the neurotransmitters _____ and _____ in the brain. Treatment of psychosis with antipsychotic medications is based on reducing the function of these neurotransmitters.

6.  In addition to the thought and neurologic symptoms, schizophrenia affects the person's abilities to relate to self and others, and to _____.

7.  Michael, 20, is brought into the clinic by his parents. They complain that during the past 6 months he has been sleeping more, avoiding friends and family, and saying "weird things to no one in particular." You realize this may be a prodromal phase before a full _____ episode.

## MULTIPLE CHOICE

Circle the answer that best completes the following statements.

1.  The negative symptoms of schizophrenia involve a deficit or decrease of normal functions and include:
    A.  volition.
    B.  increased speech.
    C.  anhedonia.
    D.  sad affect.

2.  Positive (or psychotic) symptoms seem to be an excess or distortion of normal functions and include:
    A.  hallucinations and delusions.
    B.  delusions and mania.
    C.  mania and hallucinations.
    D.  anxiety and delusions.

3. People with schizophrenia die earlier than other people do. The largest contributor to this excess mortality rate is:
   A. heart attack.
   B. suicide.
   C. cancer.
   D. renal failure.

4. The brain disorder in schizophrenia renders many affected people unable to understand that they are mentally ill. The percentage of people **NOT** receiving treatment at any given time because of lack of insight is:
   A. 90%.
   B. 40%.
   C. 54%.
   D. 11%.

5. A coexisting problem common in schizophrenia is:
   A. homelessness.
   B. anxiety.
   C. chronic disease.
   D. substance abuse.

6. For psychiatric inpatients, the therapeutic milieu should be:
   A. simple, safe, and restrictive.
   B. restrictive, flashing lights, and safe.
   C. tolerant, safe, and dependent.
   D. pleasant, simple, and safe.

7. Antipsychotic medications are used to treat disorders such as schizophrenia that are characterized by psychosis. These drugs are also called:
   A. neurostimulators.
   B. mood stabilizers.
   C. neuroleptics.
   D. anticonvulsants.

8. A young woman approaches you on the street asking for your forgiveness. She believes that you are a demon and screams loudly, "I know who you are! You talk to me all the time." You remember from your nursing class that schizophrenia may result in:
   A. craziness.
   B. delusions.
   C. denial.
   D. drinking.

9. Roger, age 28 and diagnosed with schizophrenia, stopped taking his medication. Within a year there will be what percentage of relapse with his psychosis?
   A. 80%
   B. 95%
   C. 0%
   D. 18%

10. It is important for clients on antipsychotic therapy to be assessed for abnormal involuntary movement with a scale such as:

A. AIMS.

B. MME.

C. HESI.

D. NCLEX.

## CRITICAL THINKING EXERCISE

Read the following situation. Unscramble the words and define each term. Answer the questions using the nursing process of assessment, diagnosis, planning, implementation and evaluation.

*Przhcheiianso* affects people differently. Any individual client may need to try several different *siipysttnachco* before finding the one that works well. This trial process can be *gzemnrdoaiil*. The nurse should explain this to clients, telling them that the health care provider will work with the client until the right one is found, and that no one will give up *peho*.

1. What is a major problem in the treatment of schizophrenia and why?

2. What types of medications and goal of treatment should the nurse expect?

3. Discuss EPS signs and symptoms.

# Chapter 49

## Caring for Clients with Mood Disorders

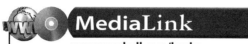

**MediaLink**

www.prenhall.com/burke

Use the address above to access the free, interactive Companion Website created for this textbook. Get hints, instant feedback, and textbook references to chapter-related NCLEX-style questions. Link to other interesting sites.

**Audio Glossary:**

Use the Companion Website, or the CD-ROM disk enclosed with your textbook, to hear the pronunciation of key terms in this chapter.

When mood goes beyond the normal range of intensity, when elation or tragedy are persistent, are not a response to life experiences, and interfere with daily functioning, a disorder of mood exists.

## MOOD DISORDERS

Match each term with its appropriate definition.

| | |
|---|---|
| 1. _____ Mood | A. Normal range of emotions |
| 2. _____ Affect | B. Inability to feel pleasure |
| 3. _____ Euthymic | C. The emotions a person is currently expressing |
| 4. _____ Hypersomnia | D. A pervasive and sustained emotion that influences how a person perceives the world |
| 5. _____ Phototherapy | E. A mental disorder |
| 6. _____ Anhedonia | F. Abnormal or excessive dilation of the pupils |
| 7. _____ Depression | G. Sleeping too much |
| 8. _____ Mydriasis | H. Light therapy |
| 9. _____ Manic speech | I. Period of persistently elevated, expansive, or irritable mood |
| 10. _____ Mania | J. Rapid and pressured |

## FILL IN THE BLANK

Fill in the blanks with the appropriate word or phrase.

1. The nurse knows that depression is not just brought about by one specific event or cause. Depression is a _____ disorder.

2. Major Depressive Disorder is _____ times more common among first-degree biologic relatives of affected people than among the general population (American Psychiatric Association, 2000).

3. The hypothalamus, pituitary, and adrenal glands, together called the _____, control the physiologic responses to stress.

4. _____ usually develops within 3 weeks after delivery. It is characterized by depressed mood, lack of concentration, guilt, lack of interest in the baby, rejection of the baby, or unreasonable fear that something bad will happen to the baby.

5. "The blues" usually starts within 3 to 4 days after delivery and lasts no longer than 2 weeks. It usually resolves without medical treatment. This is called _____.

6. _____ is thought to be a result of abnormal melatonin metabolism.

7. Because of the _____ associated with mental illness, people with depression are less likely to accept treatment, to comply with treatment recommendations, and to continue treatment than are people with general medical conditions without depression.

## MULTIPLE CHOICE

Circle the answer that best completes the following statements.

1. Diane, 30, comes into the clinic stating, "I'm so depressed!" The nurse knows that the diagnostic criteria for a major depressive episode include that the client must have at least five symptoms during:
   A. 10 days.
   B. a 2-week period.
   C. a 3-month period.
   D. 20 days.

2. A recent advance in brain imaging that shows abnormal function in the prefrontal cortex of the cerebrum and in the limbic system during depressive episodes is called:
   A. PET.
   B. CAT.
   C. EEG.
   D. PCT.

3. A major life stressor precedes the first major depressive episode for many people. The average age of onset is in the:
   A. teenage years.
   B. mid-30s.
   C. mid-20s.
   D. senior years.

4. Only 12% of people are willing to take medication for depression, while _____ would take medication for a headache:
   A. 50%
   B. 92%
   C. 36%
   D. 70%

5. The nurse knows that she must educate clients, their families, and communities about depression, its outcomes, and treatments. Knowledge can help people comply with treatment, be free from unnecessary guilt, and maintain:
   A. a healthy lifestyle.
   B. their jobs.
   C. faith.
   D. hope.

6. More Americans die each year from suicide than from homicide. An average of 85 Americans die from suicide each day. Suicide rates are highest among:
   A. older adults.
   B. children.
   C. teenagers.
   D. middle-aged adults.

7. Most antidepressants act on two major brain neurotransmitters which regulate mood:
   A. serotonin and dopamine
   B. GABA and norepinephrine
   C. serotonin and norepinephrine
   D. norepinephrine and dopamine

8. Clients tend to have better outcomes when they are treated with a combination of medications and:
   A. group therapy.
   B. psychotherapy.
   C. music therapy.
   D. cognitive therapy.

9. Unwarranted optimism, grandiosity, and poor judgment characterize:
   A. Depressive Disorder.
   B. Paranoid Disorder.
   C. Sleep Disorder.
   D. Bipolar Disorder.

10. Psychosocial factors are important in the timing of manic episodes and stressful events may precede them. Mania is a:
    A. physical condition.
    B. medicinal condition.
    C. biologic condition.
    D. mental condition.

## CRITICAL THINKING EXERCISE

Read the following situation. Unscramble the words and define each term. Answer the questions using the nursing process of assessment, diagnosis, planning, implementation, and evaluation.

While *tsssnnaatideerp* are used mostly to treat depression, there are other uses for this classification of drugs. They are used to treat *bvissseeov*-Compulsive Disorder, Panic Disorder, eating disorders, and *xtyiena* disorders. The tricyclic amitriptyline is also used as an adjunctive treatment for chronic pain. The classes of drugs used to treat *icnma* episodes are *oomd* stabilizers (antimanic agents), anticonvulsants (that act as mood stabilizers), benzodiazepines (to decrease anxiety and agitation while the other drugs are starting to work), and antipsychotics (if the client has psychotic symptoms).

1. Name the four groups of antidepressants.
2. What are the side effects of the four groups of antidepressants?
3. Discuss other forms of therapy used in conjunction with medications.

# Chapter 50

# Caring for Clients with Anxiety Disorders

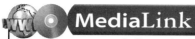

**MediaLink**

www.prenhall.com/burke

Use the address above to access the free, interactive Companion Website created for this textbook. Get hints, instant feedback, and textbook references to chapter-related NCLEX-style questions. Link to other interesting sites.

**Audio Glossary:**

Use the Companion Website, or the CD-ROM disk enclosed with your textbook, to hear the pronunciation of key terms in this chapter.

Anxiety is a normal response to stress. Everyone has experienced it. When anxiety becomes overwhelming, when it impairs a person's ability to function at home, school, or work, and affects relationships with other people, then it is a disorder. While the antianxiety medications are contraindicated as a problem-solving approach for the otherwise normal client, they are required for the well being of many people with severe Anxiety Disorders. Nurses should be aware that many people with mental disorders require medications in order to function.

## ANXIETY

Match each term with its appropriate definition.

1. _____ Anxiety
2. _____ Dysphoric
3. _____ Panic attack
4. _____ Paresthesia
5. _____ Agoraphobia
6. _____ Obsession
7. _____ Compulsion
8. _____ Phobia
9. _____ Coping
10. _____ Resilience

A.  A recurrent and intrusive thought that caused marked distress

B.  Characterized by an episode of intense fear or discomfort

C.  A feeling of uneasiness and activation of the autonomic nervous system in response to a vague, nonspecific threat

D.  The quality of being hardy or "stress resistant"

E.  Anxiety about being in places or situations where escape may be difficult

F.  A persistent and irrational fear

G.  Conscious ways that people deal with stress

H.  Repetitive behavior

I.  Uncomfortable and distressed

J.  Numbness or tingling

# FILL IN THE BLANK

Fill in the blanks with the appropriate word or phrase.

1. People experiencing Panic Disorder often visit the _____ several times before they are accurately diagnosed.

2. _____ affects three times as many women as men, and affects 1% to 2% of the general population.

3. Dorothy has come to your clinic and is in obvious distress. She states, "I need to wash my hands now! You don't know the risk I take of just being here!" You suspect Dorothy is suffering from _____.

4. The doctor ordered Klonopin 1 mg PO b.i.d. for Karen, 24, with Generalized Anxiety Disorder. You know that this drug has a _____ duration of action.

5. Jim, 32, has had difficulty sleeping for 3 months. He said he started having nightmares 3 months ago about his father, but the images are still unclear. After the nightmares he feels intense fear and hopelessness. You suspect Jim may be suffering from _____.

6. The limbic system is surrounded by the cerebral cortex. It plays a role in motivation, _____, and memory.

7. Myra tells you she is deathly afraid of crossing bridges to the point that she avoids them altogether. She doesn't visit her family because she has to cross the Golden State Bridge in order to see them. As a nurse you suspect Myra suffers from _____.

# MULTIPLE CHOICE

Circle the answer that best completes the following statements.

1. A nursing assistant catherized the wrong patient. The nurse takes her aside to point out her error. This is an example of:
   A. adaptive behavior.
   B. favoritism.
   C. maladaptive behavior.
   D. prejudice.

2. George comes to the clinic convinced he is having a heart attack. He says the symptoms started on his way to a very important job interview. You suspect George is:
   A. having case of nerves.
   B. looking for attention.
   C. having a panic attack.
   D. procrastinating.

3. To cope with anxiety by deliberately relaxing or deep breathing in situations they expect to provoke anxiety, thus interrupting the automatic anxiety responses, clients use:
   A. ACT.
   B. ADHD.
   C. CBT.
   D. CHF.

4. CBT or behavioral therapy usually takes about:
   A. 1 month.
   B. 3 years.
   C. 2 weeks.
   D. 12 weeks.

5. Mr. Tracy demonstrates frequent mood changes. These changes are termed:
   A. anxiety.
   B. labile.
   C. euphoria.
   D. depression.

6. Martha comes into the doctor's office visibly upset. You talk to her and notice that she is unaware of her anxiety. All of her VS are increased and she has pressured speech. Martha is exhibiting what level of anxiety?
   A. mild
   B. severe
   C. panic
   D. moderate

7. The limbic structure responsible for coordinating actions of the autonomic nervous system and endocrine system and involved in control of emotions, nurturing behavior, and fear conditioning is called the:
   A. hypothalamus.
   B. thalamus.
   C. amygdala.
   D. pituitary.

8. Your client has learned to verbalize his own feelings of anxiety and understand his stress response. This phase of anxiety is called:
   A. family.
   B. community.
   C. stabilization.
   D. acute.

9. Nurses can diagnose and treat the symptom of anxiety:
   A. with M.D. orders only.
   B. with health care team approval.
   C. collaboratively.
   D. independently.

10. Information about the client's usual coping methods can be helpful in:
    A. administering medicine.
    B. gaining information.
    C. discharge planning.
    D. planning care.

# CRITICAL THINKING EXERCISE

Read the following situation. Unscramble the words and define each term. Answer the questions using the nursing process of assessment, diagnosis, planning, implementation, and evaluation.

Important assessments by nurses always include how clients respond to their illnesses and how they respond to their *tmttensera*. When assessing a patient with anxiety, nurses must remember to document their *jbctveieo* findings as well as *iceetuvbsj* symptoms. *Dceesnil* nurses are also responsible for the care of clients who receive medications and must know the desired effects and potential side effects of those medications.

1. What are three nursing diagnoses related to anxiety?
2. What are the four degrees/levels of anxiety?
3. Name at least five anxiety-related disorders and five different medications along with their action.

# Chapter 51

# Caring for Clients with Personality Disorders

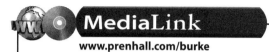

A personality disorder is an enduring pattern of inner experience and behaviors. Diagnosing personality disorders requires an evaluation of the person's long-term patterns of functioning. These clients can be manipulative, socially inappropriate, and difficult. The goal of the nurse is to provide professional care, not to be the friend of the client.

## PERSONALITY DISORDERS

Match each term with its appropriate definition.

1. _____ Personality

2. _____ Self-identity

3. _____ Impulsive

4. _____ Inflexibility

5. _____ Stern

6. _____ Linehan

7. _____ Self-invalidation

8. _____ Active passivity

9. _____ Depersonalization

10. _____ Parasuicidal

A. Behavior aimed at harming oneself

B. First used the term borderline personality in 1938

C. Includes the psychosocial traits and characteristics that make a person an individual

D. A part of normal personality development

E. Leading contemporary theorist on Borderline Personality Disorder

F. An alteration in the perception of the self in which the client feels like she is looking at herself from outside her body

G. Increasing amounts of substance needed to create an effect

H. Unable to change behavior when circumstances suggest that a change is indicated

I. Failure to recognize own emotions, thoughts, behaviors

J. Fails to work actively on solving own life problems

## FILL IN THE BLANK

Fill in the blanks with the appropriate word or phrase.

1. A person's _____ significantly affects how this person responds to life events, including illnesses.
2. The DSM-IV-TR describes _____ types of personality disorders.
3. _____ is a central problem in disorders of personality.
4. Elaine's parents report that she is misinterpreting everything they say into something that negatively affects her life. They admit this has been ongoing since she turned 10; Elaine is now 26. The nurse suspects that Elaine is using maladaptive responses in her _____.
5. _____ treatment of personality disorders is based on treating specific target symptoms rather than the disorder itself.
6. Evans, 32, is suspicious of everyone. He has difficulty obtaining and maintaining relationships. As long as no one violates his personal space he does not react violently. The nurse recognizes that Evans may be suffering from _____ disorder.
7. A cognitive deficit, such as ideas of reference, in which clients misinterpret everyday events as having a personal meaning for them, may occur in _____ disorder.

## MULTIPLE CHOICE

Circle the answer that best completes the following statements.

1. When teaching client strategies about coping with stress, the nurse uses the mnemonic Wise mind ACCEPTS. The S stands for:
   A. stimulants are great.
   B. supine position works.
   C. sensations that are intense.
   D. Serax works wonders.
2. To help people who have used self-harm for coping to find more enduring and adaptive ways to comfort themselves this technique is used:
   A. caffeine
   B. five senses exercise
   C. finger paints
   D. Valium
3. A nursing intervention for clients that have thoughts about self-harm or suicide is:
   A. negotiating a no self-harm contract.
   B. administering sedatives.
   C. allowing two visitors every 30 minutes.
   D. maintaining a dimly lit, quiet room.

4. A pervasive pattern of social shyness, feelings of inadequacy, and hypersensitivity to negative evaluation is called:
   A. Avoidant Personality Disorder.
   B. anxiety.
   C. paranoid behavior.
   D. Schizotypal Personality Disorder.

5. Mrs. Jones demonstrates a need to be taken care of. This characterizes:
   A. Dependent Personality Disorder.
   B. anxiety.
   C. Affective Disorder.
   D. depression.

6. Marsha, 38, seems overly trusting of her boss. She believes everything her boss tells her and acts on any suggestions she makes. She has alienated all her friends because of her attempts to get attention by whatever means possible. The nurse suspects that Marsha suffers from:
   A. Narcissistic Personality Disorder.
   B. Dependent Personality Disorder.
   C. an addiction.
   D. Histrionic Personality Disorder.

7. Nurses can help people with personality disorders achieve:
   A. emotional well-being.
   B. great things.
   C. personal growth.
   D. a steady income.

8. Any judgment about a client's personality must take into account that person's ethnic, social, and:
   A. monetary background.
   B. cultural background.
   C. emotional background.
   D. psychologic background.

9. A client comes to the clinic crying, "I just left my boyfriend . . . he beat me everyday, I just couldn't take it any more. I'm so weak; maybe if I could take it he would love me more." As a nurse you know the best response would be:
   A. "Are you crazy?"
   B. "If you go back, he will continue to harm you."
   C. "He is an adult and responsible for his own behavior."
   D. "Why do you want to go back?"

10. One way a nurse can prevent a client with personality disorder from disrupting the unit is by:
    A. making the unit rules clear.
    B. having a conference with staff.
    C. A and B.
    D. none of the above.

# CRITICAL THINKING EXERCISE

Read the following situation. Unscramble the words and define each term. Answer the questions using the nursing process of assessment, diagnosis, planning, implementation, and evaluation.

*Riisssictanc* Personality Disorder is characterized by a pervasive pattern of grandiosity, a need for *miirdaaton,* and a lack of *ypmetah* for others. Affected people have an inflated sense of self-importance. Treatment goals for this personality disorder include developing coping skills that involve independent problem solving without *ttxoiioepaln* of others.

1. What are the priority goals of care for this client?
2. What medications and treatments should the nurse expect to be ordered?
3. What essential information must be documented on this client's chart?

# Chapter 52

## Caring for Clients with Substance Abuse or Dependency

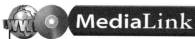

**MediaLink**

**www.prenhall.com/burke**

Use the address above to access the free, interactive Companion Website created for this textbook. Get hints, instant feedback, and textbook references to chapter-related NCLEX-style questions. Link to other interesting sites.

**Audio Glossary:**

Use the Companion Website, or the CD-ROM disk enclosed with your textbook, to hear the pronunciation of key terms in this chapter.

Substance abuse is one of the most serious health issues facing our society. The effects of substance abuse extend beyond the client to their families, friends, coworkers, and community.

## SUBSTANCE ABUSE TERMINOLOGY

Match each term with its appropriate definition.

| | | | |
|---|---|---|---|
| 1. _____ Tolerance | | A. | Staggering gait |
| 2. _____ Addiction | | B. | Exaggerated feeling of well-being |
| 3. _____ Denial | | C. | Experienced when use of a substance is discontinued |
| 4. _____ Intoxication | | D. | Symptoms caused by vitamin B deficiency |
| 5. _____ Wernicke's | | E. | Inability to remember events during intoxicated state |
| 6. _____ Ataxia | | F. | Refusal to acknowledge existence of a situation or feeling |
| 7. _____ Withdrawal | | G. | Increasing amounts of substance needed to create an effect |
| 8. _____ Blackout | | H. | Mental and physical drug-seeking behaviors |
| 9. _____ Korsakoff's | | I. | Group of reversible symptoms produced by a substance |
| 10. _____ Euphoria | | J. | Alcoholic encephalopathy |

## FILL IN THE BLANK

Fill in the blanks with the appropriate word or phrase.

1. Jennifer, age 22, reports she was sexually assaulted by her date. She cannot remember the details. The nurse suspects that Jennifer may have been given the drug _____.

2. Mr. and Mrs. Wilson discover their 17-year-old son Kyle running through the house screaming that demons are chasing him. This type of behavior may result from the use of several drugs classified as _____.

3. Mrs. Johnson is experiencing anorexia, nausea, and vomiting associated with her chemotherapy treatment. A drug that may be used to alleviate some of these symptoms is called _____.

4. A 13-year-old girl has a history of drug use that causes euphoria, loss of inhibition, and hallucinations. The substance can be found in many common household products. The nurse suspects that she might be using

   _____.

5. A college sophomore has been studying for midterm exams continuously for 24 hours. He presents to the emergency room complaining of anxiety, insomnia, and an irregular heartbeat. The drug most widely used to remain alert is

   _____.

6. Mr. Allen is hospitalized for diagnostic tests to rule out lung cancer. He has a history of smoking two to three packs of cigarettes per day. After 1 week in the hospital, Mr. Allen becomes irritable and threatens to sign out against medical advice. The nurse recognizes that Mr. Allen may be suffering from _____ withdrawal.

7. Jeremy brings his friend Kara to the emergency room following a party at his apartment. Kara is confused and complains of severe chest pain and difficulty breathing. Physical examination reveals dilated pupils, BP-168/102, P-96 irregular. The nurse knows these to be symptoms of a _____ overdose.


## MULTIPLE CHOICE

Circle the answer that best completes the following statements.

1. Drugs that distort the user's perception of reality are called:
   A. stimulants.
   B. amphetamines.
   C. hallucinogens.
   D. nicotine.

2. A medication given during alcohol withdrawal to prevent Wernicke–Korsakoff's syndrome is:
   A. caffeine.
   B. vitamin $B_1$.
   C. Dilantin.
   D. Valium.

3. A nursing intervention that provides low stimulation for the client during drug withdrawal includes:
   A. restricting visitors.
   B. administering sedatives.
   C. allowing two visitors every 30 minutes.
   D. maintaining a dimly lit, quiet room.

4. A drug prescribed to deter clients from drinking alcohol is:
   A. Antabuse.
   B. methadone.
   C. ReVia.
   D. Catapres.

5. Mr. Jones demonstrates frequent mood changes with increased alcohol intake. These changes are termed:
   A. labile.
   B. anxiety.
   C. euphoria.
   D. depression.

6. A young male increases his consumption of alcohol from one six pack to two six packs of beer per day to achieve the same effects. This action may indicate:
   A. addiction.
   B. intoxication.
   C. tolerance.
   D. dependence.

7. A local maintenance man is frequently seen drinking for hours at the local bar. He refuses to socialize with his neighbors and has been labeled an "angry man." The nurse is aware that the crucial phase of alcohol addiction includes:
   A. emotional and physical disintegration.
   B. memory blackouts.
   C. loss of control over the decision to drink or not to drink.
   D. a steady increase of alcohol consumption.

8. You remember from your nursing class that the chronic phase of alcohol addiction may result in:
   A. job loss.
   B. suicide.
   C. denial.
   D. drinking in secret.

9. A chronic alcoholic has been admitted to the medical floor for a laceration of the forehead and observation. During your physical assessment you note the presence of ascites, yellow skin, and severe muscle weakness. You suspect that this client may be diagnosed with end-stage liver disease known as:
   A. hepatic encephalopathy.
   B. alcoholic hepatitis.
   C. cirrhosis.
   D. portal hypertension.

10. A 21-year-old male was brought to the emergency room by the paramedics. They report the client was found, unresponsive, lying on a park bench. Their initial assessment noted pinpoint pupils and depressed respirations. The ER nurse suspects that this client may have overdosed on:
    A. alcohol.
    B. amphetamines.
    C. cocaine.
    D. heroin.

11. A client is concerned about the withdrawal effects from his use of the drug Ecstasy. He states, "I don't want to start shaking. I've seen it happen with my friend who drank too much." The best response by the nurse should be:
    A. "Don't worry, we'll be right here to watch you."
    B. "You won't have any withdrawal symptoms."
    C. "You should have stopped taking the drug a long time ago."
    D. "You won't have withdrawal symptoms, but you might have flashbacks."

12. At a chemical substance treatment center, the nurse is teaching the family about the importance of understanding drug withdrawal from heroin. He explains that a synthetic opiate will be used to replace the heroin. This drug is known as:
    A. methadone.
    B. naltrexone.
    C. Antabuse.
    D. Catapres.

13. You observe that the medication nurse always seems to go the bathroom after administering narcotics. You also notice that more pain medications are given when that particular nurse is on duty. Your next action should be to:
    A. do nothing; it is none of your business.
    B. confront the nurse when she comes out of the bathroom.
    C. discuss your concerns with your supervisor.
    D. continue to watch for more unusual behaviors.

14. The major goal of withdrawal management is:
    A. cessation of drug use.
    B. protection of society.
    C. physiologic safety.
    D. maintaining sobriety.

15. The nurse establishes a nursing diagnosis of Deficient Knowledge for a client during the acute phase of substance abuse treatment. Teaching should include all of the following except:
    A. consequences of drug use.
    B. reasons behind drug use.
    C. coping strategies.
    D. recommended amounts of drug use.

# CRITICAL THINKING EXERCISE

Read the following situation. Unscramble the words and define each term. Answer the questions using the nursing process of assessment, diagnosis, planning, implementation, and evaluation.

A client has been diagnosed with *horricsis* of the liver, gastrointestinal bleeding, *etiscas, nicrkewe–koffsarok* syndrome, and depression. He admits to drinking 1 to 2 pints of liquor a day and states that his last drink was before admission 3 days ago. The nurse includes monitoring for signs of *irimuled menstre* as part of the nursing care plan.

1. What are the priority goals of care for this client?
2. What medications and treatments should the nurse expect to be ordered?
3. Discuss the signs and symptoms of delirium tremens.
4. What essential information must be documented on this client's chart?

# Answer Key

## Chapter 1 The Medical–Surgical Nurse

### Matching

1. H
2. F
3. A
4. D
5. E

6. G
7. C
8. I
9. J
10. B

### Fill in the Blank

1. standards for nursing practice of LP/VNs
2. nursing process
3. teacher
4. quality assurance
5. PES
6. initial assessment
7. ANA Code for Nurses

### Multiple Choice

1. C
2. B
3. A
4. C
5. A

6. B
7. A
8. B
9. C
10. A

11. C
12. C
13. A
14. C
15. D

### Critical Thinking Exercise

**Advanced directive**—formal document that expresses the wishes of a client in the event of mental incapacitation

**Durable power of attorney**—substitute decision maker

**Advocate**—one who speaks up for another

**Ethical dilemma**—a situation in which both answers have negative or unpleasant effects

1. If client is not fed he will most likely lapse into a coma and die; if the client is fed his verbal wishes are ignored.
2. Right to make informed choices and decisions regarding his care.

3. The advanced directive has not been identified; however, the client is still mentally capable of making decisions; this request cannot be ignored by the son, doctor, or nurse.
4. Nursing actions and interventions must be documented by law.

# Chapter 2 The Adult Client in Health and Illness

## Matching

| | | | |
|---|---|---|---|
| 1. | I | 6. | B |
| 2. | D | 7. | E |
| 3. | C | 8. | J |
| 4. | G | 9. | A |
| 5. | H | 10. | F |

## Fill in the Blank

1. young adults
2. middle adult
3. old-old
4. young-old
5. middle-old
6. suicide
7. transition

## Multiple Choice

| | | | | | |
|---|---|---|---|---|---|
| 1. | A | 5. | D | 9. | B |
| 2. | B | 6. | A | 10. | C |
| 3. | A | 7. | C | 11. | D |
| 4. | D | 8. | A | 12. | D |

## Critical Thinking Exercise

**Acute**—rapid onset, lasts short period of time, self-limiting

**Substance abuse**—using a medication or drug for recreational use

**Gonorrhea**—sexually transmitted disease, may be seen in the young adult

**Pregnancy**—state of carrying a developing fetus in the uterus

1. Stage 4 entails the assuming of the dependent sick role; client may be admitted to the hospital for treatment; responses to the illness depends on the client's age, severity of illness, support systems, previous coping mechanisms.
2. Client has a history of alcohol dependency, which lowers inhibitions; substance abuse is a major concern for clients in the young adult stage; sexually active young adults who do not use condoms and have multiple sexual partners are at an increased risk of pregnancy and the transmission of STIs.

3. Chronic illnesses may be permanent and may leave a client disabled; causes nonreversible physiologic changes; may extend for years. Acute illnesses are short, rapid, and generally treatable.
4. Pregnancy test positive. Notified physician.

# Chapter 3 The Older Adult Client in Health and Illness

## Matching

1. J
2. C
3. E
4. A
5. G
6. B
7. D
8. H
9. I
10. F

## Fill in the Blank

1. gerontologic nursing
2. old-old
3. young-old
4. middle-old
5. immune theory
6. 77.7 years
7. drug reactions, interactions

## Multiple Choice

1. C
2. A
3. B
4. B
5. C
6. A
7. A
8. D
9. C
10. B

## Critical Thinking Exercise

**Aging**—progressive changes related to the passage of time

**Physical**—concerning or pertaining to the body

**Psychosocial**—related to both psychologic and social factors

**Behaviors**—the actions or reactions of an individual under specific circumstances

**Lifestyles**—pattern of living and behavior of an individual, society, or culture

1. Arthritis, hypertension, hearing and vision impairments, cardiovascular diseases, cataracts, sinusitis, orthopedic disorders, diabetes, and Alzheimer's disease.
2. Answers will vary.

3. Early detection of diseases, immunizations, injury prevention, self-management techniques. People who are physically active, eat a healthy diet, do not use tobacco, and practice other healthy behaviors reduce their risk for chronic illnesses and have half the rate of disability as those who do not.

## Chapter 4 Settings of Care

### Matching

1. B
2. I
3. C
4. H
5. D
6. E
7. J
8. F
9. A
10. G

### Fill in the Blank

1. rehabilitation process
2. adult day care facility
3. home health care
4. client safety
5. handicap
6. home care bill of rights
7. referral source

### Multiple Choice

1. C
2. D
3. D
4. B
5. C
6. D
7. B
8. D
9. A
10. A
11. A
12. B
13. D
14. B
15. D

### Critical Thinking Exercise

**Long-term care facility**—variety of institutions that provide nursing care for clients who cannot care for themselves

**Rehabilitation**—the process of restoring the ability of a person to live and work as normally as possible within his or her own limitations

**Community**—group of persons sharing common interests and needs

**Impairment**—a decrease in strength or value

1. Level of mobility, self-care ability, bowel and bladder function, mental status.
2. Mr. Elliot's frustration and despair.
3. Hopelessness—allow Mr. Elliot to verbalize his concerns, assist him to recognize the actual cause of his frustration and anger, collaborate with him to develop short-term goals.

4. Always document facts, not judgments. When possible, document the client's words in quotation marks.

# Chapter 5 Guidelines for Client Assessment

## Matching

1. D
2. I
3. B
4. F
5. E

6. A
7. C
8. G
9. H
10. J

## Fill in the Blank

1. vital signs, height, weight, hygiene, odor, posture, gait, manifestations of illness, speech, facial expression
2. cyanosis
3. pallor
4. constriction
5. diaphragm
6. Snellen
7. wheezes

## Multiple Choice

1. A
2. B
3. C
4. D
5. D

6. D
7. A
8. B
9. A
10. B

11. A
12. D
13. A
14. A
15. B

## Critical Thinking Exercise

**Manifestations**—objective and subjective data associated with specific illnesses

**Dyspnea**—difficulty breathing

**Assessment**—collection of data to identify health care needs

**Inspection**—detailed, visual examination of body part

1. Partial assessment.
2. Focused assessment.
3. Vital signs; breath sounds; respiratory effort: retraction and use of accessory muscles for breathing; sputum: amount, color, consistency; presence of edema; skin color; temperature and moisture content.
4. Client complains of SOB; pink, frothy sputum; dyspnea; and chest pain. Inspection of the chest reveals increased respirations and retraction of

intercostal muscles. Nasal flaring is noted. Lung sounds auscultated in all lung fields. Crackles heard in bases of both lungs. Cardiac sounds are muffled. Apical pulse irregular, rapid at 130 bpm. Client is anxious and states that he feels like he is going to die.

## Chapter 6 Essential Nursing Pharmacology

### Matching

| | | | |
|---|---|---|---|
| 1. | B | 6. | F |
| 2. | J | 7. | C |
| 3. | H | 8. | G |
| 4. | A | 9. | E |
| 5. | D | 10. | I |

### Fill in the Blank

1. loading dose
2. efficacy
3. ethnicity
4. synergism
5. potentiation
6. Food, Drug, and Cosmetic Act
7. Controlled Substances Act

### Multiple Choice

| | | | |
|---|---|---|---|
| 1. | C | 6. | B |
| 2. | D | 7. | C |
| 3. | A | 8. | D |
| 4. | A | 9. | C |
| 5. | B | 10. | C |

### Critical Thinking Exercise

**Administer**—to give, as in medication to a patient

**Standing**—an order (from the physician) that is standard for every patient

1. Right drug, right client, right time, right route, right dose, right documentation.
2. Wrong dose, wrong drug, and wrong route.
3. Use of only acceptable abbreviations and symbols developed by JCAHO when transcribing medication orders to the MAR.

# Chapter 7 Caring for Clients with Altered Fluid, Electrolyte, or Acid–Base Balance

## Matching

1. I
2. H
3. C
4. E
5. D
6. G
7. F
8. J
9. A
10. B

## Fill in the Blank

1. hyperkalemia
2. hyponatremia
3. hypocalcemia
4. chronic respiratory acidosis
5. metabolic acidosis
6. metabolic alkalosis
7. hypocalcemia

## Multiple Choice

1. A
2. D
3. B
4. B
5. B
6. D
7. A
8. B
9. A
10. B
11. A
12. A
13. D
14. B
15. C

## Critical Thinking Exercise

**Hypovolemia**—decrease in blood volume

**Hyponatremia**—decreased sodium in the blood

**Hypokalemia**—decreased potassium in the blood

**Electrolyte**—substances needed in the body to help regulate water, assist in enzyme reactions; plays a major role in neuromuscular activity

1. Assess respiratory status.
2. Age, large volumes of IV fluids.
3. Administration of a loop diuretic via the IV, decrease in the IV flow rate, EKG.
4. Client complains of SOB and chest pain. Vital signs: T-99, R-32, P-102, BP-162/88. Crackles noted in bilateral lower lobes, use of accessory muscles for breathing. Client is coughing up copious amounts of thick, white sputum.

# Chapter 8 Caring for Clients in Pain

## Matching

1.  E
2.  J
3.  H
4.  A
5.  F
6.  I
7.  D
8.  B
9.  C
10. G

## Fill in the Blank

1.  ice packs
2.  secondary gain
3.  cutaneous pain
4.  neuropathic pain
5.  impaired blood flow
6.  food, milk
7.  opiate

## Multiple Choice

1.  A
2.  D
3.  A
4.  B
5.  C
6.  A
7.  B
8.  C
9.  B
10. C
11. D
12. D
13. B
14. C
15. D

## Critical Thinking Exercise

**Duragesic**—trade name for fentanyl, opioid analgesic, management of chronic pain

**Transdermal**—pertaining to the transport of medication through the skin

**Relaxation**—various techniques used to reduce tension

**Patient-controlled analgesia**—use of a device that allows the patient to administer a set amount of pain medication without the risk of overdose

1.  Stop the PCA pump immediately, call for help, initiate oxygen therapy using standing orders, obtain vital signs, notify the physician.
2.  IV administration of the antidote, Narcan (naloxone), which reverses respiratory depression.
3.  Monitor vital signs at least every 15 minutes for several hours, assess LOC concurrently with the vital signs, monitor pain level, provide reassurance. Many clients who experience an overdose of a narcotic are transferred to the ICU for 24-hour observation.
4.  Found patient unresponsive to verbal and mechanical stimuli. PCA pump placed on hold and oxygen therapy 3 L/nc initiated. Vital signs T-99.4, P-16, R-8, BP-98/64. Charge nurse administered Narcan via IV. Patient aroused to verbal stimuli.

# Chapter 9 Caring for Clients Having Surgery

## Matching

1. E
2. J
3. I
4. H
5. G

6. C
7. F
8. B
9. A
10. D

## Fill in the Blank

1. preoperative
2. diaphragmatic
3. Jackson Pratt and Hemovac
4. Valium
5. lithotomy
6. surgical scrub
7. sanguineous

## Multiple Choice

1. B
2. C
3. C
4. D
5. B

6. C
7. C
8. B
9. C
10. C

11. C
12. B
13. B
14. C
15. C

## Critical Thinking Exercises

**Anesthesia**—medication used to produce loss of consciousness, loss of sensation and reflexes, muscle relaxation

**Jackson Pratt**—type of bulb device that uses suction to drain surgical wounds

**Sanguineous**—bloody drainage

**Atelectasis**—collapsed or airless lung

1. The client is agitated and restless. She also moans at times.
2. Client states that her pain is a 7 on a pain scale of 1–10. She is restless and agitated, but drowsy. Client is able to respond to questions but moans on occasion. Last dose of pain medication, morphine, was given 1 hour ago.
3. Review the pain medication orders to determine if the morphine can be given at this time. Monitor the vital signs. Attempt to use other pain relief measures, such as repositioning. Ensure that the temperature in the room is comfortable for Mrs. Fields, dim the lights and reduce the noise level as much as possible. Document your actions and notify the physician if the pain level continues to increase. Make sure that Mrs. Fields' bladder is not distended, as this will cause agitation and discomfort.
4. Risk for Injury related to effects of morphine.

# Chapter 10 Caring for Clients with Inflammation and Infection

## Matching

1. F
2. I
3. G
4. H
5. A

6. E
7. B
8. D
9. J
10. C

## Fill in the Blank

1. acute
2. systemic manifestations
3. chronic
4. inflammatory process
5. convalescent
6. nosocomial, urinary tract
7. inappropriate use of antibiotics

## Multiple Choice

1. A
2. C
3. B
4. A
5. D

6. D
7. D
8. B
9. A
10. C

11. D
12. C
13. A
14. B
15. A

## Critical Thinking Exercise

**Inflammation**—nonspecific response to an injury

**Lymphadenitis**—enlargement of the lymph nodes

**Cellulitis**—inflammation that has spread to surrounding connective tissues

**Leukocytosis**—increased WBC production

1. It would be important to contact the long-term care facility and speak with the nurse. Inquire about the fall and any pertinent information relating to risk for other injuries. Have any other residents been diagnosed with MRSA? Has this client received any other antibiotic therapy recently? Discuss his nutritional status.
2. Impaired Skin Integrity—perform wound care as ordered, administer antibiotics, monitor for signs of increased infection. Risk for Imbalanced Body Temperature—infection increases body temperature.
3. Vancomycin—observe for signs of allergic reaction and hypotension; monitor for toxicity effects, such as ringing in the ears or difficulty hearing; monitor urine output.
4. Sterile dressing performed on left lower leg. Wound approximately 5 cm in length and 2 cm in diameter. Edges not approximate with purulent drainage

noted. Area around wound red and edematous. Cleansed with sterile NS, applied sterile 2 × 2s and reinforced with 4 × 4s and kerlix. Client tolerated procedure with no pain.

## Chapter 11 Caring for Clients with Altered Immunity

### Matching

1. E
2. C
3. G
4. A
5. H

6. B
7. J
8. D
9. I
10. F

### Fill in the Blank

1. passive immunity
2. antibody titer
3. eggs
4. hypersensitivity
5. oral thrush
6. graft-versus-host disease
7. Kaposi's sarcoma

### Multiple Choice

1. C
2. C
3. D
4. D
5. A

6. A
7. C
8. C
9. C
10. A

11. B
12. B
13. B
14. C
15. C

### Critical Thinking Exercise

**AIDS**—acquired immunodeficiency syndrome

**Candidiasis**—fungus that commonly affects the mouth, respiratory tract, or vagina

**Lymphoma**—any neoplastic disorder of the lymphoid tissue

**Dysplasia**—alteration in size, shape, and organization of adult cells

1. History of recent nausea or vomiting, difficulty eating, fatigue syndrome; preferred diet.
2. Altered Nutrition, Less than Body Requirements—consult with dietitian regarding the appropriate diet, serve small, nonspicy portions of food, encourage frequent oral hygiene, monitor weight and lab results. Risk for Impaired Skin Integrity—monitor for signs of skin breakdown, obtain egg

crate mattress, sheep skin protectors, or similar items, turn every 2 hours, encourage ambulation or range-of-motion exercises.

3. Ineffective Individual Coping—assess client's support network and coping skills, provide continuity of care.

4. S: Upon admission client states, "I don't think I can handle this anymore."
O: Client tearful; history of fatigue and diarrhea.
A: Risk for ineffective coping.
P: Assess support system and promote positive coping behaviors. Suggest social worker and dietary consults.

## Chapter 12 Caring for Clients with Cancer

### Matching

| | | | |
|---|---|---|---|
| 1. | E | 6. | B |
| 2. | D | 7. | F |
| 3. | G | 8. | J |
| 4. | A | 9. | H |
| 5. | C | 10. | I |

### Fill in the Blank

1. deoxyribonucleic acid
2. Staging
3. lung
4. lung, bladder
5. marijuana
6. Chemotherapy
7. hospice

### Multiple Choice

| | | | | | |
|---|---|---|---|---|---|
| 1. | C | 6. | A | 11. | A |
| 2. | C | 7. | C | 12. | D |
| 3. | B | 8. | C | 13. | B |
| 4. | D | 9. | D | 14. | B |
| 5. | B | 10. | A | 15. | A |

### Critical Thinking Exercises

**Cancer**—group of neoplastic diseases

**Staging classification**—a method of classifying a cancer based on tumor size, node involvement, and metastasis

**Incontinent**—inability to control bowel or bladder excretion

**Nolvadex**—generic name is tamoxifen; treatment of choice for breast cancer

1. Very large tumor, metastasis to numerous lymph nodes, bone involvement.
2. Functional Urinary Incontinence.
3. Total Urinary Incontinence—apply protective barrier to perineal area, cleanse skin thoroughly after each episode. Pain—determine client's current pain medication orders, assess pain scale level and location.
4. Client states that she has lost 10 pounds in the last 2 months. Unable to eat solid foods. Frequently complains of nausea and vomiting. Taste and sense of smell are limited.

# Chapter 13 Caring for Clients Experiencing Shock, Trauma or Critical Illness

## Matching

| | | | |
|---|---|---|---|
| 1. H | | 6. E | |
| 2. I | | 7. F | |
| 3. J | | 8. B | |
| 4. G | | 9. A | |
| 5. D | | 10. C | |

## Fill in the Blank

1. hypovolemic shock
2. pneumothorax
3. massive protein loss
4. anaphylactic shock
5. early septic shock
6. penetrating
7. peritonitis

## Multiple Choice

| | | | | | |
|---|---|---|---|---|---|
| 1. D | | 6. B | | 11. B | |
| 2. B | | 7. A | | 12. D | |
| 3. A | | 8. A | | 13. B | |
| 4. D | | 9. B | | 14. C | |
| 5. C | | 10. A | | 15. D | |

## Critical Thinking Exercises

**Anxious**—worried about an uncertain event

**Pedal pulses**—arterial pulses found on the top of the foot, dorsalis pedis

**Urine output**—the amount of urine excreted from the kidneys, normal value 30 mL/hr

**Septic shock**—form of shock resulting from bacterial toxins in the bloodstream

1. Darvocet is a combination drug (propoxyphene/acetaminophen) that reduces the body temperature and controls pain. The body produces a

temperature in response to infection. Suppressing the temperature masked this response.
2. No order for a dressing change. Patient immobile due to the hip surgery. No report of the wound status noted.
3. State only facts. Need vital signs, objective and subjective data obtained during your assessment, including appearance of wound, urine output.
4. No! The lack of observation of the wound did contribute to the patient's condition. Document only facts in the chart, including your phone conversation with the physician. It is possible that an incident report may be filed in order to investigate what factors contributed to the fact that the nurses did not look at the wound nor question Mr. Jenkins' increased pain level.

## Chapter 14 Loss, Grief, and End-of-Life Care

### Matching

| | | | |
|---|---|---|---|
| 1. | H | 6. | B |
| 2. | E | 7. | D |
| 3. | A | 8. | F |
| 4. | C | 9. | I |
| 5. | G | 10. | J |

### Fill in the Blank

1. denial
2. depression
3. spirituality
4. dying person's bill of rights
5. Patient Self-Determination Act
6. euthanasia
7. collaborative

### Multiple Choice

| | | | | | |
|---|---|---|---|---|---|
| 1. | B | 6. | C | 11. | B |
| 2. | D | 7. | B | 12. | C |
| 3. | A | 8. | C | 13. | B |
| 4. | A | 9. | B | 14. | A |
| 5. | C | 10. | C | 15. | B |

### Critical Thinking Exercise

**Metastasis**—moving of cancer cells from one body part to another

**Hospice**—provides palliative and supportive care to terminally ill patients

**Advanced directives**—legal documents that provide for the health-care and financial needs of a person in the event of a catastrophic illness, disease, or death

**Living wills**—legal documents prepared by a person with a sound mind to indicate the type of medical care desired if that person becomes incapacitated

1. Pain control.
2. Thoroughly assess Mrs. Gash's physical and mental status, as well as the pain issue. Develop a collaborative plan of care that addresses the needs and perceptions of the patient.
3. Caregiver Role Strain.
4. Observable behaviors and assessment data, subjective statements made by both the patient and the husband.

# Chapter 15 The Endocrine System and Assessment

## Matching

| | | | |
|---|---|---|---|
| 1. | D | 6. | F |
| 2. | E | 7. | H |
| 3. | B | 8. | C |
| 4. | G | 9. | J |
| 5. | A | 10. | I |

## Fill in the Blank

1. diabetes insipidus
2. gynecomastia
3. exophthalmos
4. diabetes mellitus
5. goiter
6. negative feedback

## Multiple Choice

| | | | |
|---|---|---|---|
| 1. | B | 6. | A |
| 2. | B | 7. | C |
| 3. | C | 8. | C |
| 4. | B | 9. | D |
| 5. | B | 10. | A |

## Critical Thinking Exercise

**Thyrotoxicosis**—condition resulting from an excessive production of thyroid hormone

**Exophthalmos**—abnormal protrusion of the eyeball due to hyperthyroidism

**Tapazole**—inhibits thyroid hormone production

**Subtotal thyroidectomy**—partial removal of the thyroid gland

1. Hemorrhage, tetany.

2. Hemorrhage—assess dressing, particularly on the posterior side; monitor blood pressure; observe for signs of restlessness. Tetany—monitor lab values for calcium deficiency, assess for peripheral tingling of toes, fingers; maintain IV fluids as ordered for administration of calcium chloride.

3. The thyroid gland produces the thyroid hormone. Removal of the entire gland, total thyroidectomy, results in the complete lack of this hormone and clients must be maintained on a hormone substitute for the rest of their lives. Partial removal of the gland allows some hormone to be produced and reduces the amount of medication required to maintain adequate blood levels.

4. Remind the client that coughing may be contraindicated immediately postop. Deep breathing exercises assist in the inflation of the lungs, which is needed to prevent collapse. Discuss the importance of pain medications, including common side effects. Explain the presence of a bulky dressing on the neck and the importance of notifying the nurse if any respiratory difficulties arise.

## Chapter 16 Caring for Clients with Endocrine Disorders

### Matching

1. D
2. E
3. B
4. G
5. H
6. F
7. A
8. C
9. J
10. I

### Fill in the Blank

1. laryngeal nerve damage
2. acromegaly
3. exophthalmos
4. myxedema coma
5. autoimmune disorder

### Multiple Choice

1. B
2. C
3. B
4. A
5. C
6. B
7. B
8. A
9. C
10. B

### Critical Thinking Exercises

**Seizures**—sudden attacks of pain, disease, or a certain symptom

**Bradycardia**—a slow heart rate with pulse of 60 or below

**Hypothermia**—body temperature below normal range

**Thyrotoxicosis**—toxic condition caused by hyperactivity of the thyroid gland

**Emergency**—any urgent condition of the client that requires immediate medical or surgical evaluation or treatment

1. Cold temperatures, infection, surgery, trauma, tranquilizers (CNS depressants).
2. Answers will vary.
3. Treatment focuses on maintaining a patent airway, stabilizing cardiac function, improving ventilation, and increasing temperature and TH levels.

## Chapter 17 Caring for Clients with Diabetes Mellitus

### Matching

| | | | |
|---|---|---|---|
| 1. | F | 6. | G |
| 2. | H | 7. | D |
| 3. | E | 8. | B |
| 4. | I | 9. | C |
| 5. | J | 10. | A- |

### Fill in the Blank

1. pancreas
2. islets of Langerhans
3. glycogenolysis
4. osmotic diuresis
5. urine
6. dawn phenomenon
7. polyuria, polydipsia, polyphagia

### Multiple Choice

| | | | | | |
|---|---|---|---|---|---|
| 1. | A | 6. | B | 11. | A |
| 2. | B | 7. | D | 12. | A |
| 3. | C | 8. | D | 13. | C |
| 4. | A | 9. | A | 14. | C |
| 5. | A | 10. | C | 15. | A |

### Critical Thinking Exercise

**Peripheral vascular disease**—any disorder affecting blood flow through the veins or arteries distal to the heart

**Hyperglycemia**—elevated blood levels of sugar

**Antibiotics**—medications used to fight infection

**Sliding scale**—a method of determining the correct dosage of regular insulin based on a blood glucose test

1. Poor circulation, peripheral neuropathy, and slow wound healing place the client at risk for a decubitus ulcer and subsequent infection.
2. A high level of glucose in the bloodstream destroys the vessels of the microvascular system, decreasing the supply of oxygen and nutrients to the tissue.
3. Pressure on the foot will further impair circulation, making it difficult for the antibiotics to destroy the pathogenic microorganisms that invade the lesion.
4. Five units of regular insulin.

## Chapter 18 The Gastrointestinal System and Assessment

### Matching

| | | | |
|---|---|---|---|
| 1. | E | 6. | D |
| 2. | I | 7. | A |
| 3. | F | 8. | C |
| 4. | J | 9. | G |
| 5. | H | 10. | B |

### Fill in the Blank

1. over-the-counter medications (aspirin, ibuprofen, NSAIDS)
2. cardiac or lower esophageal sphincter
3. vagus nerve
4. nutrition
5. endoscope

### Multiple Choice

| | | | |
|---|---|---|---|
| 1. | A | 6. | D |
| 2. | C | 7. | C |
| 3. | B | 8. | C |
| 4. | B | 9. | D |
| 5. | D | 10. | A |

### Critical Thinking Exercise

**Abdominal ultrasound**—a diagnostic procedure that provides internal images of the abdomen

**Gastritis**—inflammation of the stomach

**Gallstones**—a concretion (usually cholesterol) formed in the gallbladder or bile ducts

**Vomiting**—ejection through the mouth of gastric contents

1. Deficient Knowledge.
2. Clear liquids to begin then advance to low-fat diet because the most common type of gallstone contains cholesterol.

3. Food and fluids are withheld 8 hours prior to procedure, a cleansing enema may be ordered, the procedure is not painful, and it may be completed in 30 minutes or less.

## Chapter 19 Caring for Clients with Nutritional and Upper Gastrointestinal Disorders

### Matching

| | |
|---|---|
| 1. J | 6. H |
| 2. C | 7. A |
| 3. F | 8. B |
| 4. E | 9. D |
| 5. G | 10. I |

### Fill in the Blank

1. stomach cancer
2. candidiasis or thrush
3. perforated bowel
4. Imbalanced Nutrition: More than Body Requirements
5. gastroscopy
6. GERD
7. protein

### Multiple Choice

| | | |
|---|---|---|
| 1. C | 6. B | 11. C |
| 2. D | 7. C | 12. C |
| 3. B | 8. C | 13. B |
| 4. B | 9. B | 14. B |
| 5. C | 10. A | 15. D |

### Critical Thinking Exercise

**Gastroscopy**—inspection of the interior of the stomach with a scope

**Gastritis**—inflammation of the stomach

*Helicobacter pylori*—bacteria that causes gastritis and stomach ulcers

**NSAIDS**—nonsteroidal anti-inflammatory drugs

1. Deficient Knowledge.
2. Explain that the client will be awake but sedated throughout the procedure, the test will take about 20 or 30 minutes, the client needs to sign a consent form, no food or water 6–12 hours before the procedure.
3. Monitor vital signs and evaluate for complications such as bleeding, back pain, SOB. Withhold all food and fluids until the gag reflex returns. Explain to the client that a sore throat is common.

4. Document client teaching and understanding of the procedure, any comments or questions that might arise during the session, status of consent form.

## Chapter 20 Caring for Clients with Bowel Disorders

### Matching

1. C
2. E
3. H
4. J
5. D
6. I
7. F
8. A
9. G
10. B

### Fill in the Blank

1. diarrhea
2. irritable bowel syndrome
3. celiac disease
4. simple appendicitis
5. gastroenteritis
6. ulcerative colitis
7. cancer

### Multiple Choice

1. C
2. A
3. B
4. D
5. C
6. A
7. D
8. B
9. C
10. C
11. C
12. A
13. B
14. C
15. B

### Critical Thinking Exercise

**Hemorrhoidectomy**—surgical removal of inflamed rectal veins

**Digital reduction**—using the fingers to push the inflamed veins into the rectum

**Sclerotherapy**—injection of a medication that will destroy or harden varicosities

**Sitz**—immersing the buttocks and perineal area into warm water with or without medication to relieve inflammation

1. Administer analgesics, sitz baths, encourage the prone position and the use of soft rubber rings.
2. Drink at least 2000 L water per day, increase dietary fiber intake, exercise in moderation.
3. Discuss the various means for pain control, including the use of analgesics; encourage the use of stool softeners; report any symptoms of bleeding, fever,

abnormal discharge from the rectum or continued pain when having a bowel movement.

4. Client lying in the side position, head in semi-Fowler's position. Vital signs stable. Anal packing in place, no bleeding noted at site. Denies pain at this time.

## Chapter 21 Caring for Clients with Gallbladder, Liver, and Pancreatic Disorders

### Matching

| | | | |
|---|---|---|---|
| 1. | G | 6. | J |
| 2. | C | 7. | F |
| 3. | E | 8. | B |
| 4. | A | 9. | H |
| 5. | I | 10. | D |

### Fill in the Blank

1. cholecystitis
2. A
3. alcoholic hepatitis
4. cirrhosis of the liver
5. hepatic encephalopathy
6. cancer
7. pancreatoduodenectomy or Whipple's

### Multiple Choice

| | | | | | |
|---|---|---|---|---|---|
| 1. | A | 6. | C | 11. | D |
| 2. | A | 7. | A | 12. | A |
| 3. | D | 8. | B | 13. | D |
| 4. | B | 9. | B | 14. | B |
| 5. | D | 10. | C | 15. | A |

### Critical Thinking Exercise

**Alcoholic hepatitis**—form of hepatitis caused by excessive alcohol intake

**Jaundice**—yellowness of skin caused by deposits of bile pigment. Bile enters the bloodstream and is excreted in the urine and stool

**Serum amylase**—enzyme that breaks down starch

**Paracentesis**—surgical puncture of a cavity for fluid removal

1. Cirrhosis.
2. Verify that informed consent has been signed. Weigh the client and obtain vital signs. Ask the client to empty his bladder.
3. Anorexia and nausea often accompany hepatitis. The meals should be small and served at least six times a day. Low-fat diets are tolerated well. Ensure

or other nutritional supplements may be ordered. Encourage the client to eat more during the day, when nausea is minimal.

4. Vital signs: T-99, P-84, R-20, BP-142/64. Client voided 350 mL of dark urine. Placed in sitting position on the side of the bed. Procedure completed by the physician. Pressure dressing applied immediately to the puncture site. Vital signs obtained. No changes. Client tolerated procedure with minimal discomfort. Specimen sent to the lab.

## Chapter 22 The Respiratory System and Assessment

### Matching

| | |
|---|---|
| 1. B | 6. A |
| 2. I | 7. E |
| 3. H | 8. F |
| 4. D | 9. C |
| 5. J | 10. G |

### Fill in the Blank

1. the cough reflex does not work if the patient is unconscious
2. Ventilation
3. chemoreceptors
4. Compliance
5. secretions
6. adventitious
7. pulse oximetry

### Multiple Choice

| | |
|---|---|
| 1. B | 6. A |
| 2. A | 7. C |
| 3. D | 8. D |
| 4. C | 9. C |
| 5. C | 10. C |

### Critical Thinking Exercise

**Life**—the state of being alive

**Respiratory**—pertaining to respiration

**Lungs**—spongy organs of respiration contained within the pleural cavity

**Bronchi**—two main branches leading from the trachea to the lungs that provide a passageway for air

**Pulmonary**—concerning or involving the lungs

1. *Ventilation* (breathing): Air moves into and out of the lungs. *External respiration:* Oxygen and carbon dioxide are exchanged between the alveoli and the

blood. *Gas transport:* Blood transports oxygen and carbon dioxide to and from the lungs and the cells of the body. *Internal respiration:* Oxygen and carbon dioxide are exchanged between the blood and the cells.

2. *Ventilation,* air movement into and out of the lungs, has two phases: *inspiration,* as air flows into the lungs, and *expiration,* when gases flow out of the lungs. The two phases make up a breath, and normally occur 12 to 20 times per minute. Inspiration lasts about 1 to 1.5 seconds; expiration lasts about 2 to 3 seconds. During inspiration, the diaphragm contracts and flattens out, and the intercostal muscles contract to increase the size of the chest cavity. The lungs stretch and their volume increases. This reduces pressure within the lungs to slightly less than atmospheric pressure. Air rushes into the lungs as a result.

3. *Airway resistance* is created by friction as gases move through the airways. Resistance is increased by airway constriction or edema, excess mucus, or by tumors that narrow the airways. As resistance increases, gas flow decreases. *Compliance* is the *distensibility* (stretchiness) of the lungs. It depends on both lung tissue and the rib cage. *Elasticity* is the tendency of lung tissue to return to its uninflated size and shape.

## Chapter 23 Caring for Clients with Upper Respiratory Disorders

### Matching

| | | | |
|---|---|---|---|
| 1. | D | 6. | A |
| 2. | B | 7. | G |
| 3. | E | 8. | C |
| 4. | I | 9. | H |
| 5. | F | 10. | J |

### Fill in the Blank

1. laryngitis
2. pharyngitis
3. tonsillitis; peritonsillar abscess/quinsy
4. acute epiglottitis
5. influenza
6. allergic rhinitis
7. sinusitis

### Multiple Choice

| | | | | | |
|---|---|---|---|---|---|
| 1. | C | 6. | D | 11. | B |
| 2. | B | 7. | B | 12. | B |
| 3. | B | 8. | C | 13. | D |
| 4. | C | 9. | C | 14. | C |
| 5. | C | 10. | D | 15. | B |

## Critical Thinking Exercise

**Ecchymosis**—round or irregular-shaped blue area on the skin created by bleeding into the tissues

**Edema**—swelling, excess fluid

**Septum**—bone that separates the nasal cavities

**Nares**—nostrils, opening into the nose cavity

1. It would be important for the nurse to obtain the patient's medical history. The details surrounding the fight should be explored. Was the patient drinking? If so, how much did he consume? What was used to hit the patient's face? A fist would cause less damage than a solid object. Was there any loss of consciousness? Were there any witnesses to the altercation? Were any drugs involved?

2. Ineffective Airway Clearance—monitor for breathing difficulties, obtain pulse oximeter readings for oxygen saturation, maintain suction equipment, observe for bleeding, check and monitor cough reflex, observe for any changes in level of consciousness. Risk for Infection—trauma to the face and soft tissues increases the chance of bacteria entering the brain cavity, monitor vital signs at least every 4 hours, administer antibiotics as ordered. Alcohol is a central nervous system sedative and may cause respiratory depression and death. The combination of alcohol and other drugs may prove fatal, thus the importance of a thorough history. Pain medication will also decrease respirations. Caution is needed if medications must be given before the alcohol is excreted from the body via the liver. The patient is also at risk for falls due to the influence of the alcohol and the trauma to the face.

3. Check for spinal fluid in the ears and nose; place the patient on bed rest in the semi-Fowler's position; observe for constipation immobility, pain, and dehydration.

4. Patient is resting in semi-Fowler's position. Nasal packing intact with small amount of bloody drainage. Demerol 50 mg IM given for pain.

## Chapter 24 Caring for Clients with Lower Respiratory Disorders

### Matching

1. C
2. H
3. F
4. J
5. G

6. E
7. D
8. A
9. B
10. I

### Fill in the Blank

1. huff coughing
2. elasticity
3. flail chest

4. chronic bronchitis
5. *pneumocystis carinii*
6. aspiration pneumonia
7. asthma

## Multiple Choice

| | | | | | | | | |
|---|---|---|---|---|---|---|---|---|
| 1. | D | | 6. | D | | 11. | A |
| 2. | D | | 7. | D | | 12. | A |
| 3. | C | | 8. | D | | 13. | C |
| 4. | C | | 9. | B | | 14. | C |
| 5. | D | | 10. | A | | 15. | A |

## Critical Thinking Exercise

**Spontaneous pneumothorax**—weakened area on the lungs that allows air to enter pleural cavity

**Dyspnea**—shortness of breath

**Cyanotic**—a bluish condition of the skin caused by a reduction of hemoglobin

**Tension pneumothorax**—air escapes into the pleural cavity, causing a mediastinal shift

1. Notify the charge nurse immediately. Elevate the head of the bed. Provide support. Monitor airway and circulation.
2. Chest tube placement.
3. Vital signs, breath sounds, chest tube drainage system, insertion site, comfort level.
4. Risk for Infection.

# Chapter 25 The Cardiovascular System and Assessment

## Matching

| | | | | |
|---|---|---|---|---|
| 1. | A | | 6. | G |
| 2. | E | | 7. | J |
| 3. | F | | 8. | H |
| 4. | I | | 9. | D |
| 5. | C | | 10. | B |

## Fill in the Blank

1. less than 1 lb.
2. parietal, visceral
3. chordae tendinae
4. cardiac muscle
5. ions
6. stroke volume
7. Cardiac reserve

*Multiple Choice*

1. A
2. C
3. C
4. B
5. D

6. C
7. A
8. A
9. D
10. D

*Critical Thinking Exercise*

**Electrocardiogram**—a record of the electrical activity of the heart

**Dysrhythmias**—an abnormal or disturbed rhythm

**Myocardial**—of, or pertaining to, the heart

**Continual**—unchanging, constant

**Intermittent**—suspending activity at intervals; coming and going

1. Stress electrocardiography, pharmacologic stress testing, continuous cardiac monitoring (telemetry, Holter monitoring), sonography (Doppler studies, echocardiography), transthoracic echocardiogram (TTE), transesophageal echocardiogram (TEE), stress echocardiogram, vascular ultrasound (Doppler imaging, duplex scans).
2. Answers may vary: changes in heart rate, rhythm, or quality, changes in bp, bruising, chest pain, heart burn, thinning of hair and nails, etc.
3. Answers may vary: Pain, Decreased Cardiac Output, Ineffective Tissue Perfusion, etc.

# Chapter 26 Caring for Clients with Coronary Heart Disease and Dysrhythmias

*Matching*

1. C
2. G
3. I
4. A
5. E

6. B
7. F
8. D
9. J
10. H

*Fill in the Blank*

1. acute myocardial infarction (AMI)
2. left ventricle
3. atherosclerosis
4. Prinzmetal's
5. PTCA
6. MI
7. dysrhythmias

## Multiple Choice

| | | | |
|---|---|---|---|
| 1. | B | 6. | D |
| 2. | C | 7. | B |
| 3. | B | 8. | A |
| 4. | C | 9. | B |
| 5. | D | 10. | B |

## Critical Thinking Exercise

**Heart**—the chambered muscular organ in vertebrates that pumps blood received from the veins into the arteries, thereby maintaining the flow of blood through the entire circulatory system

**Circulation**—movement in a circle or circuit, especially the movement of blood through the body's vessels as a result of the heart's pumping action Sinoatrial—the SA node (SA stands for sinoatrial) is one of the major elements in the cardiac conduction system, the system that controls the heart rate

1. A cardiac dysrhythmia is a disturbance or irregularity in the electrical system of the heart. Cardiac dysrhythmias may be benign or life threatening. Changes in heart rhythm occur due to "normal" events such as exercise or fear, as well as to pathologic changes. Any dysrhythmia can affect cardiac output. The effect of the dysrhythmia determines the need for treatment.
2. Determine rate, determine regularity, assess P waves, assess P to QRS relationship, measure PR interval and QRS complex, identify abnormalities.
3. Answers will vary: normal sinus rhythm, sinus tachycardia, sinus bradycardia, premature atrial contractions, atrial flutter, atrial fibrillation, premature ventricular contractions, ventricular tachycardia, ventricular fibrillation, first-degree AV block, second-degree AV block, third-degree AV block.

# Chapter 27 Caring for Clients with Cardiac Disorders

## Matching

| | | | |
|---|---|---|---|
| 1. | I | 6. | C |
| 2. | E | 7. | F |
| 3. | G | 8. | A |
| 4. | B | 9. | H |
| 5. | J | 10. | D |

## Fill in the Blank

1. friable
2. Myocarditis
3. pericarditis

4. paradoxical pulse
5. cardiac tamponade
6. Pericardiocentesis
7. right-sided heart failure

## Multiple Choice

| | | | |
|---|---|---|---|
| 1. | C | 6. | D |
| 2. | C | 7. | C |
| 3. | A | 8. | B |
| 4. | B | 9. | A |
| 5. | B | 10. | C |

## Critical Thinking Exercise

**Endocardium**—endothelial membrane that lines the chambers of the heart

**Bacteria**—one-celled organisms without a true nucleus; nonpathogenic; live on skin and mucous membranes

**Mitral**—cardiac valve between the left atrium and left ventricle

**Intravenous**—within the vein

**Tricuspid**—the valve between the right atrium and right ventricle

1. Endocarditis is frequently classified by its onset and disease course. *Acute endocarditis* has an abrupt onset and is a rapidly progressive, severe disease. *Staphylococcus aureus* is the usual infective organism in acute endocarditis. In contrast, *subacute endocarditis* has a more gradual onset. It is more likely to occur in clients with preexisting heart disease. *Streptococcus viridans* is the most common organism causing subacute endocarditis.

2. Infective endocarditis generally causes elevated temperature (above 101.5°F or 39.4°C) and flulike symptoms. The client may have a cough, shortness of breath, and complain of joint pain. Acute staphylococcal endocarditis presents with sudden and more severe manifestations, including a high fever. Heart murmurs are common. Peripheral manifestations of endocarditis may include *petechiae* (small, purplish-red spots) on the trunk, conjunctiva, and mucous membranes; *splinter hemorrhages* (red streaks under the fingernails or toenails); small, painful growths on the fingers and toes; or small, purplish-red lesions on the palms of the hands and soles of the feet. Complications of infective endocarditis include heart failure, and infarctions of other organs (lungs, brain, kidneys, or bowel) from embolization of vegetative fragments.

3. Organisms in the bloodstream attach to the endocardial lining of the heart and become enmeshed in deposits of fibrin and platelets. This covering "protects" the bacteria from quick removal by the immune system. These vegetations develop on heart valve leaflets, varying in size and shape. *Friable* (easily broken, fragile) vegetations can break off, traveling through the bloodstream to other organs. When they lodge in small vessels, they may

cause hemorrhages, infarcts, or abscesses. The vegetations prevent normal valve closure, causing regurgitation of blood through the valve and heart murmurs.

## Chapter 28 Caring for Clients with Peripheral Vascular Disorders

### Matching

| | | | |
|---|---|---|---|
| 1. | E | 6. | I |
| 2. | F | 7. | H |
| 3. | D | 8. | G |
| 4. | C | 9. | J |
| 5. | A | 10. | B |

### Fill in the Blank

1. essential hypertension
2. malignant hypertension
3. intermittent claudication
4. Buerger's disease
5. Raynaud's phenomenon
6. abdominal aortic aneurysm
7. deep venous thrombosis (DVT)

### Multiple Choice

| | | | | | |
|---|---|---|---|---|---|
| 1. | A | 6. | B | 11. | A |
| 2. | C | 7. | C | 12. | A |
| 3. | C | 8. | D | 13. | A |
| 4. | D | 9. | B | 14. | D |
| 5. | C | 10. | A | 15. | B |

### Critical Thinking Exercise

**Saphenous vein**—longest vein in the body, extends down the entire leg

**Doppler ultrasonic flow test**—noninvasive test that assists in the visualization of the major vessels; used to detect abnormalities

**Angiographic**—pertaining to the use of x-rays to visualize blood vessels

**Vein stripping**—procedure used to ligate and tie off affected veins

1. Varicose veins—incompetent valves.
2. Prolonged standing, age; pregnancy.
3. Venous ulcers.
4. Assess peripheral circulation, apply antiembolic stockings, assist in passive and active range of motion on the lower extremities, elevate the extremities

# Chapter 29 The Hematologic and Lymphatic Systems and Assessment

## Matching

1. C
2. F
3. G
4. B
5. D

6. J
7. H
8. E
9. I
10. A

## Fill in the Blank

1. 10 days
2. vessel spasm, formation of platelet plug, clot formation, clot retraction, clot dissolution
3. return excess lymph to heart, remove foreign matter from lymph, filter blood and store platelets
4. pallor, cyanosis
5. complete blood count (CBC)
6. clotting study or coagulation profile
7. bone marrow study

## Multiple Choice

1. C
2. C
3. D
4. A
5. A

6. B
7. B
8. A
9. C
10. D

## Critical Thinking Exercise

**Oxygen**—a gas used medicinally to manage respiratory distress, myocardial infarction, shock, and various other lung diseases

**Nutrients**—foods or liquids that supply the body with the necessary chemicals for metabolism

**Substances**—the matter from which any organ or tissue is composed

**Cells**—protoplasm containing nuclei or nuclear materials

**Waste**—excreted material

1. Normocytic, microcytic, macrocytic, normochromic, hypochromic.
2. Sixty to 80%; three types: (1) Neutrophils are *phagocytic,* responsible for engulfing and destroying foreign matter. (2) Eosinophils make up 1% to 3% of WBCs. Their numbers increase during allergic reactions and during infestations with parasites. (3) Basophils make up 0.3% to 0.5% of total WBCs and are believed to be a part of the hypersensitivity and stress responses.
3. Lymphocytes account for 20% to 30% of WBCs. Although they are small and nondescript, lymphocytes are the primary effectors and regulators of

specific immune responses. *B lymphocytes (B cells)* are involved in forming antibodies, whereas *T lymphocytes (T cells)* take part in cell-mediated immunity. A third type of lymphocyte, *natural killer cells (NK cells),* also provides immune surveillance and resistance to infection.

# Chapter 30 Caring for Clients with Hematologic and Lymphatic Disorders

## Matching

1. C
2. H
3. I
4. B
5. G

6. D
7. A
8. J
9. F
10. E

## Fill in the Blank

1. ulcer
2. Epstein–Barr
3. Non-Hodgkin's lymphoma
4. Reed–Sternberg
5. Chemotherapy
6. Pruritis, night sweats
7. Anemia

## Multiple Choice

1. A
2. D
3. D
4. C
5. C

6. C
7. B
8. B
9. A
10. D

## Critical Thinking Exercise

**Malignant**—a growth or condition that resists treatment

**Support**—something that assists in maintenance

**Infection**—disease caused by microorganisms (most commonly bacteria)

**Lymphocytes**—white blood cells in the body responsible for immunity

**Nutritional**—foods and liquids required by the body that aid in growth, repair, and maintenance

1. Answers may vary.
2. Answers may vary.
3. If the disease is advanced, total nodal irradiation may be done. This may cause permanent sterility.

# Chapter 31 The Urinary System and Assessment

## Matching

| | |
|---|---|
| 1. D | 6. I |
| 2. C | 7. G |
| 3. F | 8. J |
| 4. H | 9. A |
| 5. E | 10. B |

## Fill in the Blank

1. 300–500
2. urethra
3. blood pressure
4. 95%, 5%
5. dehydration
6. pyuria
7. clean-catch specimen

## Multiple Choice

| | |
|---|---|
| 1. C | 6. C |
| 2. C | 7. A |
| 3. B | 8. B |
| 4. D | 9. C |
| 5. C | 10. A |

## Critical Thinking Exercise

**Contrast medium**—a substance used in radiology to fill hollow organs or blood vessels to highlight their structure

**Filtered**—liquid passed through any porous substance that prevents particles of a certain size to pass through

**Kidneys**—pair of organs in the retroperitoneal area that form urine

**Ureters**—tubes that carry urine from the kidneys to the bladder

**Renal**—pertaining to the kidney

1. KUB, intravenous pyelography (IVP), retrograde pyelography, computed tomography (CT) scan, magnetic resonance imaging (MRI), renal scan (kidney scan), ultrasound, cystoscopy.
2. Assess and clarify understanding of the procedure. Inquire about allergies to seafood, iodine, or x-ray contrast media. Notify the physician or radiologist of any known allergies. Verify signed consent for the procedure. Instruct or administer preprocedure laxatives as ordered. Allow clear liquids only for 8 hours before the test. After IVP, monitor vital signs and urinary output. Report signs of reaction to contrast media such as dyspnea, tachycardia,

itching, hives, or flushing. Check injection site for redness, pain, and warmth. Apply warm packs to the site if indicated. Increase fluid intake after the test is completed.
3. Answers may vary: Deficient Knowledge, Impaired Urinary Elimination, Fear, Anxiety, etc.

# Chapter 32 Caring for Clients with Renal and Urinary Tract Disorders

## Matching

1. C
2. E
3. A
4. G
5. I
6. B
7. J
8. D
9. H
10. F

## Fill in the Blank

1. stress incontinence
2. functional incontinence
3. benign prostatic hypertrophy
4. cystitis
5. diabetic nephropathy
6. urolithiasis
7. hydronephrosis

## Multiple Choice

1. C
2. C
3. B
4. A
5. C
6. C
7. D
8. D
9. A
10. A

## Critical Thinking Exercise

**BUN**—blood urea nitrogen

**Serum creatinine**—nitrogen compound found in the blood

**Azotemia**—presence of BUN and creatinine in the blood

**Furosemide**—generic name for Lasix, a loop diuretic used for renal disease

1. Chronic renal failure.
2. Renin produced in the kidney helps in the regulation of the blood pressure; damaged kidneys are unable to produce renin efficiently; there is an increased risk of hypertension.
3. Excess Fluid Volume and Risk for Infection.

4. The kidneys are not able to effectively remove nitrogenous waste products due to the failure of the filtration mechanisms; nitrogenous wastes are formed by the catabolism of protein; azotemia will result; and destructive systemic reactions will occur.

# Chapter 33 The Reproductive System and Assessment

## Matching

1. A
2. D
3. E
4. G
5. F

6. B
7. I
8. J
9. H
10. C

## Fill in the Blank

1. erection
2. HDL
3. Androgens
4. cervix
5. bacteriostatic
6. presenting problem
7. diethylstilbestrol

## Multiple Choice

1. C
2. D
3. B
4. A
5. C

6. D
7. C
8. A
9. B
10. D

## Critical Thinking Exercise

**Structures**—arrangement of component parts in organisms

**Reproductive**—pertaining to reproduction, the process by which plants and animals produce offspring

**Functions**—actions performed by any organism

**Pleasure**—the feeling of being pleased or delighted

**Sexual**—pertaining to sex or having sex

1. Spermatogenesis takes 64 to 72 days, and includes the following processes: Sperm stem cells *(spermatogonia)* divide to produce daughter cells *(spermatocytes)* that have the same number of chromosomes (46) as the parent cell. Spermatocytes further divide to produce *spermatids,* immature cells with half the number of chromosomes (23) as the spermatocyte. Spermatids mature

into sperm cells with a head and a tail. The head contains enzymes that allow the sperm to penetrate and fertilize the ova. The tail allows the sperm to move. When the sperm and ova fuse, the resulting cell has the normal number of chromosomes (46).

2. The menstrual cycle begins at the onset of menstruation. During the *menstrual phase,* the inner endometrial layer detaches and is expelled as menstrual fluid. As the maturing follicle begins to produce estrogen, the *proliferative phase* begins. The inner endometrial layer is repaired and thickens, while spiral arteries proliferate and tubular glands form. Cervical mucus becomes thin, helping sperm move into the uterus. During the *secretory phase,* progesterone increases endometrial vascularity and prepares it to support the fertilized ovum. Cervical mucus thickens, blocking the internal os. If fertilization does not occur, hormone levels fall. Spasm of spiral arteries causes degeneration and sloughing of the inner endometrial layer, starting the process again.

3. *Colposcopy* is used to examine tissues of the vagina and cervix using a brightly lighted microscope. Colposcopy can identify early premalignant changes in cervical tissue, and is performed when Pap test results are abnormal. This procedure usually is accompanied by *endocervical curettage* to obtain cell samples for examination and biopsy. Colposcopy should be scheduled early in the client's menstrual cycle (between days 8 and 12). This invasive procedure requires informed consent. Instruct the client to avoid using any vaginal creams or medications prior to the procedure. The client is placed in lithotomy position during the procedure. Tell the client that she will feel a pinch or momentary cramping sensation when the specimen is obtained. Provide psychologic support, because this procedure often is performed when an abnormal Pap smear result has been obtained. Instruct the client to refrain from sexual intercourse or insertion of anything into the vagina (e.g., tampons) until the cervix has healed, approximately 7 to 10 days.

## Chapter 34 Caring for Male Clients with Reproductive System Disorders

### Matching

1. D
2. G
3. E
4. C
5. I

6. J
7. H
8. B
9. F
10. A

### Fill in the Blank

1. benign prostatic hyperplasia
2. prostatitis
3. prostate cancer
4. cryptorchidism
5. testicular torsion
6. hydrocele
7. vasectomy

## Multiple Choice

| | | | | | |
|---|---|---|---|---|---|
| 1. | D | 6. | C | 11. | B |
| 2. | B | 7. | A | 12. | B |
| 3. | A | 8. | A | 13. | C |
| 4. | B | 9. | B | 14. | A |
| 5. | A | 10. | D | 15. | D |

## Critical Thinking Exercise

**Cryptorchidism**—failure of one or both of the testes to descend into the scrotum

**Alpha fetoprotein**—protein produced by some cancers, used to monitor the effectiveness of cancer treatments

**Lactic dehydrogenase**—tumor marker; elevated levels may indicate testicular cancer

**Ultrasound**—noninvasive diagnostic procedure used to detect soft tissue damage

1. Chemotherapy combined with surgery, followed by radiation therapy.
2. Assess the client's current level of sexual function, reinforce teaching on the effects of surgery on sexual function, discuss possibility of saving sperm in a sperm bank, allow the client to grieve and express concerns.
3. Information regarding regular testicular examinations; knowledge of complications that should be reported to the physician; pain medication usage, including side effects. Teaching should reflect the type of treatment for the cancer. Discussion of returning to sexual activity should also be initiated.
4. Document surgical site to include dressing and wound care, vital signs, activity level, diet, and intake and output.

# Chapter 35 Caring for Female Clients with Reproductive System Disorders

## Matching

| | | | | |
|---|---|---|---|---|
| 1. | B | 6. | H |
| 2. | D | 7. | J |
| 3. | F | 8. | I |
| 4. | A | 9. | G |
| 5. | E | 10. | C |

## Fill in the Blank

1. fibrocystic breast changes
2. mastitis
3. premenstrual syndrome
4. primary dysmenorrhea
5. menopause

6. cystocele
7. endometriosis

## Multiple Choice

| | | | | | |
|---|---|---|---|---|---|
| 1. | D | 6. | A | 11. | B |
| 2. | B | 7. | C | 12. | C |
| 3. | D | 8. | A | 13. | A |
| 4. | A | 9. | D | 14. | B |
| 5. | B | 10. | C | 15. | B |

## Critical Thinking Exercise

**Invasive carcinoma**—condition in which cancer cells have spread to the surrounding tissues

**Peau d'orange**—dimpled skin condition seen in breast cancer

**Nipple retraction**—inversion of the nipple

**Breast-conserving surgery**—removing the tumor, surrounding tissue, and several lymph nodes; may be followed by radiation treatments

1. Decisional Conflict: Treatment Options
2. Discuss the disease process and options. Provide an opportunity for the client to ask questions. Make eye contact if culturally acceptable. Answer questions simply and honestly.
3. Reinforce preoperative teaching and routine postoperative care, including pain control, wound care, activity restrictions, diet, special equipment, such as a JP drain, and IV fluids.
4. Nurse's notes should contain all of your teaching points to include the client's acknowledgment of understanding and any questions that might arise during the session.

# Chapter 36 Caring for Clients with Sexually Transmitted Infections

## Matching

| | | | |
|---|---|---|---|
| 1. | G | 6. | I |
| 2. | E | 7. | B |
| 3. | H | 8. | A |
| 4. | F | 9. | C |
| 5. | J | 10. | D |

## Fill in the Blank

1. chlamydia
2. genital herpes
3. genital warts
4. gonorrhea

5. syphilis
6. prostatitis
7. latency

## Multiple Choice

| | | | | | |
|---|---|---|---|---|---|
| 1. | A | 6. | A | 11. | D |
| 2. | B | 7. | D | 12. | D |
| 3. | D | 8. | A | 13. | D |
| 4. | D | 9. | B | 14. | B |
| 5. | D | 10. | D | 15. | B |

## Critical Thinking Exercise

**Intercourse**—any physical contact between two individuals with the stimulation of the genital organs of at least one

**Chlamydia**—STI caused by a gram-negative organism; can cause scarring in the uterine tubes if left untreated

**Gonorrhea**—highly contagious STI caused by the *Neisseria gonorrhoeae* bacteria

**Cefotetan**—trade name for a second-generation cephalosporin; used in the treatment of pelvic inflammatory disease

1. Cervical discharge culture during a Pap test.
2. Syphilis and possibly HIV.
3. Did the client complete her medication regime? Has the client kept all of her follow-up appointments? Is the client able to discuss ways to prevent future STI occurrences? Is she engaging in safer sex practices?
4. Anxiety—emphasize that most STIs can be treated effectively. Discuss the possible transmission of any STI to the newborn child. Impaired Social Interaction—explain that STIs are behavior problems. STIs are not punishment and can be prevented.

# Chapter 37 The Nervous System and Assessment

## Matching

| | | | |
|---|---|---|---|
| 1. | E | 6. | J |
| 2. | D | 7. | H |
| 3. | B | 8. | I |
| 4. | C | 9. | A |
| 5. | G | 10. | F |

## Fill in the Blank

1. SNS, PNS
2. optic nerve

3. corneal reflex
4. hearing balance
5. level of consciousness
6. nystagmus
7. reflexes

## Multiple Choice

| | | | |
|---|---|---|---|
| 1. | D | 6. | C |
| 2. | A | 7. | D |
| 3. | B | 8. | B |
| 4. | C | 9. | B |
| 5. | A | 10. | C |

## Critical Thinking Exercise

**Brain**—nerve tissue housed within the cranium of the skull

**Nervous**—pertaining to the nerves

**Skull**—bony structure of the head (8 cranial bones, 14 facial bones, and the teeth)

**Malfunctions**—defective actions performed by organisms

**Disorders**—pathologic conditions of the mind or body (disease)

1. (1) Dura mater, the outer layer; (2) arachnoid, the middle layer; and (3) pia mater, the inner layer directly attached to the brain.
2. Cerebrum, diencephalon, brainstem, and cerebellum.
3. The brain receives about 750 mL of blood each minute and uses approximately 20% of the body's cardiac output. This large oxygen demand is necessary for glucose metabolism, which is the brain's only source of energy. The brain cannot store oxygen or glucose so it needs a constant supply of both. Two arterial systems supply blood to the brain: (1) internal carotid arteries and (2) vertebral arteries. Most of the cerebrum is supplied blood by the internal carotid arteries. The brainstem and cerebellum receive their blood supply from the vertebral arteries. These major arteries are connected by smaller arteries forming a ring called the *circle of Willis*. This circle protects the brain by providing alternative blood flow routes when an artery is blocked. Cerebral veins drain venous blood into the jugular veins.

# Chapter 38 Caring for Clients with Intracranial Disorders

## Matching

| | | | |
|---|---|---|---|
| 1. | H | 6. | C |
| 2. | J | 7. | A |
| 3. | I | 8. | G |
| 4. | B | 9. | D |
| 5. | E | 10. | F |

## Fill in the Blank

1. meningitis
2. corticosteroid
3. spinal fluid
4. encephalitis
5. neglect syndrome
6. dysarthria
7. epidural hematoma

## Multiple Choice

| | | | | | |
|---|---|---|---|---|---|
| 1. | B | 6. | C | 11. | A |
| 2. | B | 7. | A | 12. | D |
| 3. | D | 8. | B | 13. | C |
| 4. | C | 9. | D | 14. | B |
| 5. | D | 10. | B | 15. | C |

## Critical Thinking Exercise

**Expressive aphasia**—the patient understands written and spoken words but cannot say what they mean

**Disarthria**—speech difficulty due to muscle damage

**Hemiplegia**—paralysis on one side of the body

**Streptokinase**—medication used to break down clot formations

1. Age, history of CHF, hypertension, and IDDM. The CVA could have occurred before the fall down the stairs.
2. Suction the airway, if necessary. Position the client in the side-lying position or high-Fowler's. Monitor respiratory status. Do not feed until a swallowing test has been completed.
3. The CVA possibly was caused by a clot lodging in the brain. The medication will break down the old clot and prevent new clots from forming.
4. Present health status; changes in memory; sudden severe headaches; difficulty speaking or understanding the spoken word; any visual changes; feelings of dizziness, numbness, tingling or facial, leg, or arm weakness; difficulty walking or loss of balance; bowel or bladder incontinence.

# Chapter 39 Caring for Clients with Degenerative Neurologic and Spinal Cord Disorders

## Matching

| | | | | |
|---|---|---|---|---|
| 1. | D | 6. | G |
| 2. | J | 7. | A |
| 3. | E | 8. | B |
| 4. | I | 9. | F |
| 5. | H | 10. | C |

## Fill in the Blank

1. spinal fusion
2. Guillain–Barré syndrome
3. trigeminal neuralgia
4. S1–S5
5. Bell's palsy
6. rabies
7. tetanus

## Multiple Choice

| | | | | | |
|---|---|---|---|---|---|
| 1. | A | 6. | B | 11. | C |
| 2. | B | 7. | B | 12. | D |
| 3. | D | 8. | B | 13. | D |
| 4. | B | 9. | C | 14. | A |
| 5. | A | 10. | A | 15. | D |

## Critical Thinking Exercise

**Alzheimer's**—irreversible senile dementia

**Aricept**—anticholinesterase drug that improves memory and reasoning in 40% of Alzheimer's patients

**Electroencephalogram**—study of brain wave patterns

**Magnetic resonance imaging scan**—a magnetic scanner used to show brain size

1. Short-term memory loss, forgetfulness with attempts to cover up the memory loss, difficulty learning new information or making decisions, decreased concentration ability, may become angry or depressed.
2. Face the client directly when speaking; use simple sentences.
3. Encourage self-care as much as possible, demonstrate use of equipment when necessary, assist with bathing as needed, help to lay out clothing, encourage fluids, limit choices.
4. Present health status and objective data such as angry outbursts and lapses in memory.

# Chapter 40 Caring for Clients with Eye and Ear Disorders

## Matching

| | | | | |
|---|---|---|---|---|
| 1. | A | 6. | J |
| 2. | H | 7. | F |
| 3. | I | 8. | D |
| 4. | E | 9. | C |
| 5. | B | 10. | G |

## Fill in the Blank

1. presbyopia
2. cataracts
3. glaucoma
4. otitis media
5. presbycusis
6. myringotomy
7. Meniere's disease

## Multiple Choice

| | | | | | |
|---|---|---|---|---|---|
| 1. C | | 6. D | | 11. B | |
| 2. B | | 7. D | | 12. B | |
| 3. C | | 8. B | | 13. A | |
| 4. A | | 9. C | | 14. A | |
| 5. A | | 10. C | | 15. D | |

## Critical Thinking Exercise

**Presbyopia**—diminished ability of the lens to accommodate as a person ages

**Entropion**—inversion of the margin of the eyelid

**Glaucoma**—group of diseases characterized by increased intraocular pressure

**Conjunctivitis**—inflammation of the conjunctiva usually caused by a virus or bacteria

1. Eyedrops are the most common treatment; they are used to decrease pressure in the eye. Laser surgery may also be used.
2. Meticulous hand washing and avoid rubbing the eyes.
3. Ask client to describe signs and symptoms of eye discomfort, changes in vision. Use of corrective lenses; obtain past medical history information, including medications.
4. Client complains of itchy, dry, and scratchy eyes. States having difficulty reading. No complaints of pain. No significant medical history noted.

# Chapter 41 The Musculoskeletal System and Assessment

## Matching

| | | | |
|---|---|---|---|
| 1. F | | 6. H | |
| 2. E | | 7. A | |
| 3. J | | 8. D | |
| 4. I | | 9. G | |
| 5. B | | 10. C | |

## Fill in the Blank

1. periosteum
2. hormones
3. synovial fluid (or bursae)
4. internal mechanism
5. lactic acid
6. height
7. falls

## Multiple Choice

1. B
2. A
3. C
4. B
5. A

6. C
7. B
8. C
9. B
10. A

## Critical Thinking Exercise

**Synovial**—pertaining to the synovia, the lubricating fluid of the joints

**Cartilage**—dense connective tissue that can withstand considerable tension; has no nerve or blood supply of its own

**Fibrous**—thread-like or film-like structures

**Cavity**—a hollow space

**Fluid**—nonsolid, liquid, or gaseous substance

1. The three primary types of joints are:
   Synarthrosis—immovable joints (e.g., such as skull sutures)
   Amphiarthrosis—slightly movable joints (e.g., vertebral joints)
   Diarthrosis or synovial—freely movable joints (e.g., shoulders, hips).
2. Ligaments are bands of connective tissue that connect bones to bones. Ligaments either limit or enhance movement, provide joint stability, and enhance joint strength. Tendons are fibrous connective tissue bands that connect muscles to bones and enable the bones to move when skeletal muscles contract.
3. Skeletal muscle, also known as voluntary muscle, allows voluntary movement. Both smooth muscle and cardiac muscle are involuntary; their movement is controlled by internal mechanisms. The muscles of the bladder wall, gastrointestinal system, and bronchi are smooth muscle. Cardiac muscle is in the heart.

## Matching

| | | | |
|---|---|---|---|
| 1. | J | 6. | H |
| 2. | C | 7. | F |
| 3. | G | 8. | B |
| 4. | I | 9. | E |
| 5. | A | 10. | D |

## Fill in the Blank

1. fat emboli
2. compartment syndrome
3. deep venous thrombosis
4. femoral head necrosis
5. carpal tunnel syndrome
6. phantom limb pain
7. contractures

## Multiple Choice

| | | | |
|---|---|---|---|
| 1. | C | 6. | B |
| 2. | D | 7. | B |
| 3. | B | 8. | A |
| 4. | C | 9. | B |
| 5. | A | 10. | C |

## Critical Thinking Exercise

**Compound fracture**—broken bone protrudes through the skin, increasing the risk for infection

**ORIF**—open reduction internal fixation; uses screws, plates, pins, nails, or wires to mend broken bones

**Neurovascular check**—assessment of sensation and circulation distal to a fracture

**Fat embolism**—fat globules from the yellow bone marrow enter the bloodstream and migrate to the lungs, potentially causing blockage of the vessels

1. Neurovascular checks—involve assessing skin color, temperature, sensation, movement, presence of edema, and capillary refill in the extremities.
2. Risk for Ineffective Tissue Perfusion, Impaired Physical Mobility, and Deficient Knowledge.
3. Chest pain, petechiae on the skin and mucous membranes, respiratory distress.
4. Alert and oriented to person, place, and time. Leg elevated on two pillows. Toes pink and warm to touch. Moves toes without difficulty. Sensation to touch acknowledged by client. Noted 2-cm area of red drainage on anterior

surface of cast. Denies pain at present time. Lungs clear bilaterally. Oxygen saturation at 98% room air. IV 1000 mL Ringer's lactate 125 mL/hour infusing in left arm.

## Chapter 43 Caring for Clients with Musculoskeletal Disorders

### Matching

1. E
2. F
3. G
4. H
5. D

6. I
7. B
8. C
9. A
10. J

### Fill in the Blank

1. scoliosis
2. systemic lupus erythematosus
3. gout
4. osteoarthritis
5. osteoporosis
6. osteomyelitis
7. plasmaphoresis

### Multiple Choice

1. A
2. D
3. C
4. A

5. C
6. C
7. D
8. D

9. B
10. D
11. A
12. B

### Critical Thinking Exercise

**Osteoarthritis**—degenerative joint disease related to wear and tear on the joints

**Crepitus**—grating sound caused by rubbing of bone on bone

**Arthroplasties**—plural for arthroplasty; repair or replacement of a joint

**Acetaminophen**—used for mild to moderate pain and fever

1. Teach active and passive ROM. Teach good body mechanics. Encourage rest periods. Teach the use of canes or walkers, if prescribed.
2. Acetaminophen serves as an analgesic, but has no anti-inflammatory properties.
3. Teach Mary about the use of the overhead trapeze. Discuss postoperative pain control. Teach the use of the incentive spirometer, coughing, and deep breathing.

4. Document vital signs, neurovascular checks, amount and color of drainage in the suction device, condition of dressing to knees, intake and output, and pain level.

# Chapter 44 The Integumentary System and Assessment

## Matching

1. E
2. D
3. H
4. I
5. B
6. G
7. J
8. C
9. F
10. A

## Fill in the Blank

1. integumentary
2. dermis
3. carotene
4. sweat
5. cerumen
6. xerosis
7. erythema

## Multiple Choice

1. C
2. D
3. A
4. B
5. C
6. C
7. A
8. D
9. D
10. B

## Critical Thinking Exercise

**Skin**—largest organ of the body; covers the outer surface

**Tissue**—collection of similar cells and their intracellular components that perform a specific function

**Elasticity**—being able to be stretched and return to original shape

**Turgor**—normal tension in a cell

**Hypothermia**—body temperature below 35° Celsius (95°F)

1. Answers may vary: dry, itchy skin; hyperpigmentation; skin tags; coarse, thin hair; gray hair; nails thick and yellow.
2. Overall production of melanocytes decreases, while abnormal localized proliferations of melanocytes may occur in specific areas. This localized hyperpigmentation may lead to the development of senile lentigines, commonly called "liver spots." These flat, brown macules commonly appear on the arms

and hands in areas of sun exposure. Keratoses also result from hyperpigmentation. Seborrheic keratoses are dark, raised lesions. Actinic keratoses are reddish, raised plaques on areas of high sun exposure. They may become malignant.

3. Both hair and nail growth decrease with aging. Older men may develop coarse hair in the ears and nose and over the eyebrows. Decreased estrogen levels may cause postmenopausal women to develop dark facial hair over the upper lip and under the chin. Hair becomes gray due to a reduction of melanocytes. Nails may thicken, yellow, and peel.

## Chapter 45 Caring for Clients with Skin Disorders

### Matching

| | | | |
|---|---|---|---|
| 1. | F | 6. | H |
| 2. | J | 7. | I |
| 3. | D | 8. | A |
| 4. | G | 9. | E |
| 5. | B | 10. | C |

### Fill in the Blank

1. Pruritis
2. Psoriasis
3. Contact or allergic
4. Exfoliative
5. acne
6. vulgaris
7. abruptly

### Multiple Choice

| | | | |
|---|---|---|---|
| 1. | A | 6. | D |
| 2. | B | 7. | A |
| 3. | C | 8. | C |
| 4. | C | 9. | B |
| 5. | B | 10. | C |

### Critical Thinking Exercise

**Psoriasis**—chronic, recurrent skin disease characterized by bright red macules covered with silvery scales

**Herpes simplex II**—acute viral disease, lesions are present on the lips, nares, or genitals

**Condylomata acuminata**—venereal warts

**Pressure ulcers**—ulcer due to local interference in circulation

1. Turn every 2 hours, support extremities with pillows/foam wedges, keep skin lubricated, decrease pressure on bony areas, and use lifting techniques to reposition.
2. Maintain Standard Precautions; use gloves when washing perineal area.
3. Topical medication for psoriasis—Tazorac gel; topical medication for herpes simplex II—acyclovir.
4. Skin intact and moist with the exception of lesions noted on the tip of the penis. Patches of silvery scales are observed on both elbows and the left knee.

## Chapter 46 Caring for Clients with Burns

### Matching

1. F
2. D
3. G
4. I
5. A
6. H
7. J
8. B
9. C
10. E

### Fill in the Blank

1. burn shock
2. acquired immunodeficiency
3. carbon monoxide
4. Curling's ulcer
5. 30–50 mL/hour
6. pulse oximeter
7. rule of nines

### Multiple Choice

1. C
2. D
3. C
4. C
5. A
6. B
7. A
8. A
9. C
10. A
11. D
12. A
13. B
14. D
15. C

### Critical Thinking Exercise

**Hydrotherapy**—"whirlpooling"; method of removing burned tissues to induce healing

**Debridement**—removal of necrotic tissue

**Silvadene**—topical anti-infective used to prevent infection in second- and third-degree burns

**Escharotomy**—surgical incision into the burned tissue to allow the return of blood flow

1. 63%.
2. Renal failure, infection, fluid overload.
3. Monitor respiratory status, monitor intake and output, monitor for signs of infection, maintain comfort.
4. Documentation of Foley catheter insertion, complete physical assessment data, wound care.

# Chapter 47 Mental Health and Assessment

## Matching

1. D
2. F
3. A
4. C
5. H
6. G
7. I
8. B
9. J
10. E

## Fill in the Blank

1. echolalia
2. serotonin
3. cope
4. body image
5. describe yourself in five words, how do you feel about yourself?
6. two-thirds
7. depression

## Multiple Choice

1. B
2. B
3. C
4. A
5. D
6. D
7. C
8. B
9. A
10. C

## Critical Thinking Exercise

**Psychologic**—pertaining to the science dealing with mental processes and their effects on behavior

**Functioning**—performing an action

**Initial**—the first as in an "initial" exam

**Assessment**—an appraisal or evaluation of a client's condition by a physician or nurse

**Facility**—an institution capable of providing care to clients

1. Psychologic functioning—thinking, feeling, behavior, response to current stressors. Social functioning—relationship with self and others and community support.
2. Because they affect each person's health attitudes and behaviors related to health and illness.
3. Culture is the attitudes, beliefs, customs, and behaviors that are passed from one generation to the next. Culture influences how we dress, what we eat, what work we do, our religion, language, customs, family roles, parenting behavior, the way we relate to other people, how we educate our children, our values, attitudes about right and wrong, and the priorities we set for our lives.

## Chapter 48 Caring for Clients with Psychotic Disorders

### Matching

1. C
2. B
3. J
4. A
5. E
6. F
7. I
8. D
9. H
10. G

### Fill in the Blank

1. Schizophrenia
2. cognitive
3. electrical activity
4. December through April
5. dopamine, norepinephrine
6. function in society
7. psychotic

### Multiple Choice

1. C
2. A
3. B
4. B
5. D
6. D
7. C
8. B
9. A
10. A

### Critical Thinking Exercise

**Schizophrenia**—a thought disorder characterized by delusions, hallucinations, disorganized speech and behavior, flat affect, and social withdrawal

**Antipsychotics**—medications given to control symptoms of schizophrenia and other kinds of psychiatric disorders

**Demoralizing**—behavior destructive of morale and self-reliance

**Hope**—the expectation that something desired will occur

1. Medication compliance is a major problem for clients with schizophrenia. It can also create problems for nurses in the psychiatric setting, especially when clients do not believe that they are sick. Approximately 80% of those who stop taking their medication after an acute episode will have a relapse of psychosis within a year. Even people who continue to take their medications experience relapse at the rate of approximately 30% in a year. Medication clearly improves the quality and quantity of life for people with severe mental illnesses such as schizophrenia. Unfortunately, the people who need medications the most often do not realize this. Also, certain medications cause side effects that combine with lack of insight to further decrease client compliance.

2. The antipsychotics are grouped as either typical (first generation), atypical (second generation), or new generation antipsychotic drugs. The goals of treatment with antipsychotic agents are to relieve symptoms of psychosis, provide for safety, and improve clients' functioning and quality of life.

3. While antagonism of $D_2$ receptors causes a reduction in psychosis, it also causes extrapyramidal side effects (also called EPSE or EPS for extrapyramidal symptoms). EPS result from the effects of antipsychotic drugs on the extrapyramidal tracts of the central nervous system, which control involuntary movement. EPS are very uncomfortable for clients. When a client experiences EPS, the provider may reduce the dose of the antipsychotic, prescribe a different antipsychotic medication, or try an anticholinergic or other medication to treat the symptoms. Anticholinergic medications are usually given orally, but some may be given intramuscularly in emergent situations. It is the responsibility of the nurse to ask whether the client is uncomfortable and to advocate for the client to obtain relief.

## Chapter 49 Caring for Clients with Mood Disorders

### Matching

1. D
2. C
3. A
4. G
5. H

6. B
7. E
8. F
9. J
10. I

### Fill in the Blank

1. multifactoral
2. 1.5 to 3
3. HPA axis
4. Postpartum psychosis
5. postpartum depression
6. Seasonal Affective Disorder or SAD
7. stigma

## Multiple Choice

1. B
2. A
3. C
4. D
5. D

6. A
7. C
8. B
9. D
10. C

## Critical Thinking Exercise

> **Antidepressants**—any medication or therapy used to prevent, cure, or alleviate mental depression
>
> **Obsessive**—excessive in degree or nature
>
> **Anxiety**—a state of apprehension, uncertainty, and fear resulting from the anticipation of a realistic or fantasized threatening event or situation, often impairing physical and psychologic functioning
>
> **Manic**—mood state characterized by excessive energy, poor impulse control, psychosis, agitation, etc.
>
> **Mood**—a pervasive emotion that influences a person's perception of the world

1. Tricyclic antidepressants (TCAs) and related cyclic agents, selective serotonin reuptake inhibitors (SSRIs), monoamine oxidase inhibitors (MAOIs), and other antidepressants (also called the *novel antidepressants*) such as Wellbutrin, Effexor, Serzone, Remeron.

2. The cyclic compounds have more side effects than the SSRIs and other miscellaneous antidepressants. As a group the tricyclics tend to cause sedation, orthostatic hypotension, weight gain, and anticholinergic side effects.

   The SSRIs have less severe anticholinergic, cardiovascular, and sedating side effects than the TCA or MAOI antidepressants but they still do cause these effects for some clients. They have a higher incidence of sexual side effects (decreased libido, ejaculatory and orgasmic dysfunction) than the TCAs. They also have more GI effects, such as nausea, loose stools, and weight loss.

   MAOI drugs can cause hypertensive crisis when combined with other drugs, and foods containing tyramine. Symptoms of hypertensive crisis are a throbbing headache, sense of speeding or pounding heart, and stiff neck.

3. Psychotherapy, cognitive therapy, behavior therapy, interpersonal psychotherapy, moderate physical exercise, electroconvulsive therapy (ECT).

# Chapter 50 Caring for Clients with Anxiety Disorders

## Matching

1. C
2. I
3. B
4. J
5. E

6. A
7. H
8. F
9. G
10. D

## Fill in the Blank

1. emergency room
2. Panic Disorder
3. OCD or Obsessive-Compulsive Disorder
4. long
5. PTSD or Post-Traumatic Stress Disorder
6. emotion
7. gephyrophobia

## Multiple Choice

1. A
2. C
3. C
4. D
5. B

6. B
7. C
8. C
9. D
10. D

## Critical Thinking Exercise

**Treatments**—any specific procedure used to cure or alleviate symptoms of disease or condition

**Objective**—visible or tangible perceptions (external)

**Subjective**—perceptions of internal origin

**Licensed**—official or legal permission granted to perform professional actions in a specific field

1. Anxiety, Ineffective Coping, Post-Trauma Syndrome.
2. Mild, moderate, severe, panic.
3. Generalized Anxiety Disorder, Panic Disorder with or without Agoraphobia, Agoraphobia without Panic Disorder, Obsessive-Compulsive Disorder (OCD), Acute Stress Disorder, Post-Traumatic Stress Disorder, Anxiety Disorder due to a general medical condition, Substance-Induced Anxiety Disorder.
   Benzodiazepines are CNS depressants. They enhance the effects of gamma-aminobutyric acid (GABA), which is an inhibitory neurotransmitter:

alprazolam (Xanax), chlordiazepoxide (Librium), clonazepam (Klonopin), clorazepate (Tranxene), diazepam (Valium), lorazepam (Ativan). Nonbenzodiazepine sedative hypnotics: zolpidiem (Ambien), temazapam (Restoril).

# Chapter 51 Caring for Clients with Personality Disorders

## Matching

1. C
2. G
3. D
4. H
5. B

6. E
7. I
8. J
9. F
10. A

## Fill in the Blank

1. personality
2. eleven
3. Impaired self-identity
4. thinking patterns
5. Pharmacologic
6. Paranoid Personality
7. Schizotypal Personality

## Multiple Choice

1. C
2. B
3. A
4. A
5. A

6. D
7. C
8. B
9. C
10. C

## Critical Thinking Exercise

**Narcissistic**—the act of loving and admiring oneself

**Admiration**—to have a high opinion of; esteem or respect

**Empathy**—identification with and understanding another's situation, feelings, and motives

**Exploitation**—utilization of another person or group for selfish purposes

1. Cognitive-behavioral therapy helps many people, but it takes time, commitment, and insight on the part of the client. Many people with personality disorders lack the insight to realize that they have a problem. Personality traits of "agreeableness" and "conscientiousness" tend to make people more responsive to therapy for disorders of personality.

2. Pharmacologic treatment of personality disorders is based on treating specific target symptoms rather than the disorder itself. Antidepressants and mood-stabilizing drugs are often used to treat symptoms of depression of mood lability. Antipsychotic drugs may be useful if a client experiences psychosis, which is occasionally a symptom in severe situations.

3. Collect subjective and objective data about the client's mental status (see Chapter 47 about mental status assessment). Observe and describe the client's verbal and nonverbal behavior objectively in the chart. Pay particular attention to the client's anxiety level. Ask about medications the client takes at home. Document statements that indicate the client's thought processes.

# Chapter 52 Caring for Clients with Substance Abuse or Dependency

## Matching

| | | | |
|---|---|---|---|
| 1. | G | 6. | A |
| 2. | H | 7. | C |
| 3. | F | 8. | E |
| 4. | I | 9. | D |
| 5. | J | 10. | B |

## Fill in the Blank

1. Rohypnol
2. hallucinogens
3. marijuana
4. inhalants
5. caffeine
6. nicotine
7. cocaine

## Multiple Choice

| | | | | | |
|---|---|---|---|---|---|
| 1. | C | 6. | C | 11. | D |
| 2. | B | 7. | C | 12. | A |
| 3. | D | 8. | B | 13. | C |
| 4. | A | 9. | C | 14. | C |
| 5. | A | 10. | D | 15. | D |

## Critical Thinking Exercise

**Cirrhosis**—end stage of liver disease, liver cell damage, and destruction

**Ascites**—abnormal fluid accumulation in the abdominal cavity

**Wernicke–Korsakoff syndrome**—alcoholic encephalopathy that results from a deficiency of vitamin $B_1$ and severe malnutrition

**Delirium tremens**—group of symptoms associated with withdrawal from alcohol

1. Physiologic safety, including relief of respiratory distress, prevention of hemorrhage, prevention of cardiovascular collapse. Improve nutritional status. Provide psychological support. Promote prevention of self-injury.
2. IV thiamine, paracentesis, insertion of a Blakemore tube, administration of sedatives such as Librium, and nutritional support such as TPN.
3. Confusion, hallucinations, anxiety, belligerent behavior, hypertension, tachycardia, tachypnea, tremors.
4. Vital signs every 2 to 4 hours, respiratory status, abdominal girth, intake and output, behavioral changes, signs of bleeding, tolerance/response to treatments.